The Alzheimer's Medical Advisor

A Caregiver's Guide to
Common Medical and
Behavioral Signs and
Symptoms in Persons
with Dementia

Philip D. Sloane, MD, MPH

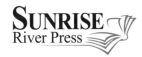

Sunrise River Press
838 Lake Street South
Forest Lake, MN 55025
Phone: 651-277-1400 or 800-895-4585
Fax: 651-277-1203
www.sunriseriverpress.com

Editor: Philip D. Sloane, MD, MPH.

Contributors: Anna Beeber, PhD, GNP, RN; Lisa P. Gwyther, MSW; Christine Lathren, MD, MSPH; Bobbi Matchar, MSW; Philip Sloane, MD, MPH; and Sheryl Zimmerman, PhD.

Student Researchers and Co-Authors: Nainisha Chintalapudi, Samuel Dotson, Jennifer Dove, Dean Fox, Jamie Hughes, Laura James, Kaleb Keyserling, Peter Marcinkowski, Erin McGillicuddy, Geoff McGowen, Disha Miyani, Lindsay Morris, Hannah Noah, Sarah Owens, Brendan Payne, Hillary Rouse, and Christopher Schifeling.

Caregiver Advisory Panel: Joe Clark, Gloria Dewey, Betty Frei, Maggi Grace, Kathy LaFone, Carol Land, Joan Peluso, Lynette Russell, and Hongly Truong.

Book design: Kenesson Design, Inc.

Development was supported in part by grant #R01 NR014199-01 from the National Institute for Nursing Research.

ISBN 978-1-934716-66-3
Item No. SRP666

Library of Congress Cataloging-in-Publication Data

Names: Sloane, Philip D., author.

Title: The Alzheimer's medical advisor : a caregiver's guide to common medical and behavioral signs and symptoms in persons with dementia / Philip Sloane, MD, MPH, Anna Beeber, PhD, GNP, RN, Sheryl Zimmerman, PhD, Christine Lathren, MD, MSPH, Lisa P. Gwyther, MSW, Bobbi Matchar, MSW.

Description: Forest Lake, MN : Sunrise River Press, 2017.

Identifiers: LCCN 2017010145 | ISBN 9781934716663

Subjects: LCSH: Dementia~Nursing~Handbooks, manuals, etc. | Dementia~Patients~Care~Handbooks, manuals, etc.

Classification: LCC RC521 .S585 2017 | DDC 616.8/310231~dc23

LC record available at https://lccn.loc.gov/2017010145

Written, edited, and designed in the U.S.A.
Printed in China
10 9 8 7 6 5 4 3 2

Table of Contents

This book is dedicated to the millions of family members, friends, neighbors, and professionals who provide care and support to persons with Alzheimer's disease and related conditions. We hope the knowledge and skills gained from this book will help you become a more confident caregiver.

Introduction

As we get older, most of us at one time or another will need help from family or friends because of a medical condition. If the condition is temporary, the need for help is short-lived—for example, after a hospitalization or a broken bone. Chronic conditions, however, require long-term, ongoing assistance.

Alzheimer's disease and other dementias are such a condition. They require care that is ongoing for a long time, usually many years. In addition, there are several unique things about the care needs of someone with dementia:

- The condition and the type and amount of assistance needed change over time.
- Problems with thinking and memory lead to new, different, and often challenging behaviors.
- Care needs include medical problems, such as signs and symptoms like cough, pain, and swelling.
- It's sometimes difficult to know when a medical problem is present, because people with dementia can't always express their feelings in words.

Even with these challenges, caregivers who use this book can learn to recognize signs and symptoms and make informed decisions, thereby providing better care and feeling less stressed. It was developed by experts from the University of North Carolina at Chapel Hill and Duke University, based on the latest clinical knowledge and scientific research. Contents include:

- basic facts about Alzheimer's disease and other dementias;
- tips on taking care of yourself while taking care of someone else;
- two-page guides about the most common problems and situations families must address when providing care;
- instruction on how to better decide whether someone is sick, in pain, or dehydrated;
- practical guidance when conferring with health care providers; when visiting hospitals, nursing homes, and assisted living residences; and during the dying process; and
- recording sheets and checklists to help organize yourself.

How to Use This Book

Begin by familiarizing yourself with each section of the book. Some chapters will be relevant to your situation now, others may inform future situations and decisions. You may decide to read cover to cover, or you may skip around according to your current needs. In any case, the skills you'll gain by reviewing Chapter 6—Keeping an Eye on Medical Issues and General Health—are important for all situations.

The guidance provided in Chapter 5 is problem-specific. For problems you encounter frequently, review the relevant guide; you may want to bookmark pages for reference. Any time you encounter a new problem, be sure to check the book for guidance. You may also find it useful to review guides for potential problems that might occur, as a way to increase your confidence and be prepared for unknown future situations. Research has found that people who use this resource become more confident about handling medical issues.

The recording sheets at the end of the book can be photocopied or torn out for use. Remember to have them handy as you communicate with health care providers.

About Alzheimer's Disease and Other Dementias

Everyone is in the same boat...
or maybe in a different boat, but
on the same river.

*— Maggi G., about being
a caregiver to someone
living with dementia*

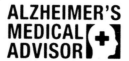

About Alzheimer's Disease and Other Dementias

Dementia is a brain disease that damages brain cells and causes the person to lose memory and other thinking skills. This damage can affect the person's ability to remember and do everyday things, as well as their behavior, mood and personality.

Causes of Dementia

Dementia has many causes; the most common are displayed in the table below. Because there is no blood test for dementia, and symptoms of different types of dementia overlap, it is sometimes hard for doctors to figure out which type of dementia a person has. Alzheimer's disease is the most common diagnosis. "Mixed" dementia is also common—it means a person shows signs of more than one kind of dementia.

Common Causes of Dementia in Older Persons

Diagnosis	Percent of Dementias	Cause	Common Early Signs
Alzheimer's disease	60%–70%	Unknown. Partly due to heredity. Vascular disease can make it worse.	Slow development of thinking problems over months to years, usually starting with forgetting things that happened recently or trouble learning new things.
Vascular dementia	10%–20%	Many small strokes, usually occurring over years.	Problems with thinking or behavior happen suddenly, seem to get better for a while, and then worsen, with the pattern happening over and over.
Fronto-temporal dementia	5%	Heredity seems to play a role, but much is unknown about its cause.	Changes in behavior or personality, such as losing interest in fun activities, or acting or speaking in ways that are unusual for the person (and may embarrass family).
Lewy body dementia	15%–25%	Unknown. Chemical changes occur in the brain that are similar to Parkinson's disease.	Trouble paying attention, problems sleeping (including moving while dreaming), seeing things that aren't there, and shaking of hands or head.
Delirium	Not a true dementia, but often mistaken for dementia	Infection, dehydration, drugs, blood chemistry imbalances, or another medical problem. Usually gets better once the problem is treated.	Quick development over days to weeks of some or all of these signs: confusion, trouble paying attention, trouble speaking, being sleepy or restless, seeing things that are not there.

Symptoms of dementia usually develop slowly and worsen over time, so they may go unrecognized for months or even years. Once a memory or other thinking problem is suspected, the doctor will often ask detailed questions (to measure various brain functions), do a physical exam, draw blood, and obtain a CAT or MRI scan. A diagnosis may take several visits over many months.

Common Changes in Persons with Dementia Over Time

Dementia is progressive—over time the brain becomes more damaged and the person has more trouble thinking and doing everyday activities. But because each person is different, it's impossible to know exactly which problems will be most severe or how quickly the person will get worse.

To know what to expect, it's helpful to think about three stages: early, mid-stage and advanced. The table below describes these stages. Of course, some people may have certain problems earlier, later, or not at all, and the time in each stage can differ for each person.

Characteristics of the Three Stages of Dementia

	Duration	Common Care Issues
Early Dementia	2-5 years	• Forgets things or recent conversations • Says things or asks questions over and over • Can no longer do complex everyday tasks, such as paying bills, shopping for groceries, or driving to a new location • Has trouble making decisions or doesn't want to try new things • Gets confused in the middle of a conversation or struggles to find words • No longer wants to do things that used to be enjoyable • Does things that seem unusual and careless, like giving away money
Mid-Stage Dementia	2-10 years	• Needs reminders or help with things like eating, bathing, dressing and using the bathroom • Forgets people and places, even those known well, and easily gets lost • Acts angry or scared, or seems to "snap" at those around them • Has trouble sleeping; may wake up at night confused • Begins to have urine and/or bowel accidents • May move slowly or shakily
Advanced Dementia	2-6 years	• Loses the ability to move around, talk, and even swallow • Requires a protective pad or pull-up because of urine and/or bowel movements • Is very confused, and has angry or sad outbursts when someone is trying to provide help • Doesn't understand words but may still enjoy calm music or soft touch

In early dementia, changes may be subtle and can sometimes be mistaken for stress or getting older. In mid-stage dementia, the changes in the person's thinking, abilities and behavior are obvious, and they need help from others to do everyday things and to stay safe. In advanced dementia, the person depends on others for nearly everything and may spend time in assisted living or a nursing home.

As dementia progresses, family caregivers need to take an increasingly larger role in making decisions about all aspects of life. At first, they need to help with things like paying bills, taking care of the house, and helping the person avoid making bad decisions. Later on, people with dementia need help with bathing and dressing. Eventually, they may no longer control their bladder and may have trouble walking. If they live long enough, a person with dementia often ends up unable to speak, unable to walk, and needing help with all daily activities. They may also lose weight because they've lost the desire to eat or drink.

The Family Caregiver's Increased Role in Managing Medical and Other Problems

As dementia progresses, the person will lose their ability to understand what is happening to them and to make decisions for themselves. As a result, family caregivers—meaning you—need to make more decisions about what you see and what needs to be done. You must observe the person carefully for clues that something is changing or is wrong. Medical professionals call these clues symptoms and signs.

Symptoms are things the person tells you about; **signs** are things you observe. Pain, dizziness, and nausea—things you can't see—are examples of symptoms. Blood pressure, temperature, a rash, or a bruise after a fall—things a caregiver can observe—are signs. In reality, there's a lot of overlap. For example, if someone with dementia suddenly gets angry about some minor thing, it is definitely a sign, but it is probably also a symptom (perhaps of anxiety). So, in this book, we mainly use the word symptom.

In dementia care, we usually talk about two general types of symptoms: medical symptoms and behavioral symptoms. Chapter 5 provides guidance for dealing with some of the most common medical and behaviorial symptoms.

- **Medical symptoms** are things such as cough, chest pain, an injury, a rash, or losing control of one's urine. In persons with dementia, they are often—but not always—caused by something other than the dementia. When a caregiver observes a symptom, they need to figure out whether it's serious or not, and what to do about it.

- **Behavioral symptoms** are things such as getting anxious or agitated, yelling, hitting a caregiver, or withdrawing and staying in bed. They often are caused by confusion, fright, or anxiety, and it seems the person is reacting (because of their brain disease) in a way that is not considered "normal." However, sometimes behavioral symptoms are caused by medical illness. This is especially true in persons with dementia who cannot explain how they feel. So, caregivers have to act a bit like a detective to determine the cause.

How to Help a Person with Dementia Stay as Healthy and Happy as Possible

At all stages of dementia, taking good care of the entire body is important, because the brain lives in the body, and if the body is healthy, the brain will be healthier. Here are things that help maintain health, prevent complications, and slow down the progression of dementia:

- Keeping high blood pressure under control
- Taking proper care of other medical conditions, such as diabetes and arthritis
- Keeping the body and teeth clean
- Getting exercise every day
- Keeping the mind active
- Doing things that involve being around others and having fun
- Being with people who give loving care

In early dementia, it's important that the person stay active and do what they enjoy as much as possible, with the help of others who can keep them safe. For example, although driving may not be safe, a family member or friend could take them to their usual activities. Having someone to talk with about fears or anger is also very important, and outings or gatherings with others who have early stage disease (with or without spouses or other family) can be helpful.

In mid-stage dementia, help with everyday living becomes more important. Because sleep problems, safety issues and behavioral symptoms are common, doctors and therapists can give advice for changes to the living space, medicines, and to the way caregivers talk and react. It's also important to remember that the person with dementia has feelings and still wants to be useful and included. Finding activities that they enjoy and can safely be a part of—like listening to music or cooking simple recipes together—often makes a big difference.

In advanced dementia, family members have to decide how to best keep their relative comfortable, and what to do if and when the person has a medical problem like an infection. Often, care needs are so great that families need paid help, or a decision is made to move to assisted living or a nursing home. Near the end of life, hospice is often helpful.

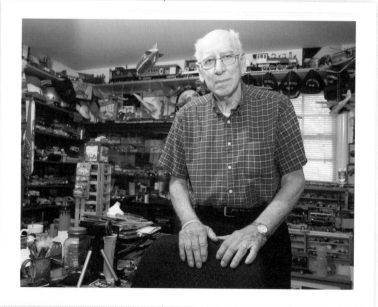

Changes in early dementia can start small and can be mistaken for stress or getting older, sometimes for years.

Where Families Caring For Someone with Dementia Can Find Help

Caring for someone with dementia can be physically and emotionally stressful. This book covers many of the key issues that family members face. There are many other helpful resources as well. The person's health care provider is a good place to start in finding resources. In addition, every county or region of the country has professionals who can provide guidance, such as the local Area Agency on Aging or the Alzheimer's Association. Support groups exist in most communities to help caregivers compare notes with others who are having similar experiences. Chapter 3 in this book provides additional advice for caregivers around relieving stress.

National Dementia Organizations

Alzheimer's Association
1-800-272-3900
24 hours/7 days
www.alz.org
Find information to enhance care and support for persons living with Alzheimer's disease and related dementias and their caregivers.

The Association for Frontotemporal Dementia
1-866-507-7222
www.theaftd.org
Find information to improve the quality of life of people affected by frontotemporal degeneration and support their caregivers.

Lewy Body Dementia Association
1-800-539-9767
www.lewybodydementia.org
Find information to support people with Lewy body dementia, their families and caregivers.

Other Caregiver Support and Service Organizations

Alzheimer's Disease Education and Referral Center
1-800-438-4380
www.nia.nih.gov/alzheimers
Find information and the latest research on dementia from the National Institutes of Health.

Benefitscheckup.org
www.benefitscheckup.org
Find programs that can help pay for medicines, health care and more.

Eldercare Locator
1-800-677-1116
www.eldercare.gov
Find local community resources by entering your zip code.

Family Caregiver Alliance
1-800-445-8106
www.caregiver.org
Find resources for caregivers nationwide.

Longtermcare.gov
www.longtermcare.gov
Find information on locating and paying for long-term care.

Veterans Administration Caregiver Support
1-855-260-3274
www.caregiver.va.gov
Find resources for caregivers of veterans.

> Remember to laugh and keep a sense of humor...it's easier said than done, but it helps.
>
> — *Kathy L., caregiver*

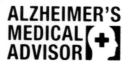

Caring for and Living with Someone with Dementia

Caring for a family member with Alzheimer's disease or another dementia involves problem solving, patience, sensitivity, and self-sacrifice. Dementia slowly robs the person of abilities they've had for all of adulthood, creating needs that the caregiver must fill or find help to fill. Dementia often also changes the personality and behavior of the person with the illness.

Yet throughout the entire illness, the caregiver recognizes that some of that person they always knew remains, which makes caregiving especially personal, but also bittersweet. And through it all, the caregiver goes forward not knowing exactly what will happen from day-to-day or over the long run.

That's because dementia can express itself in many different ways, and so each caregiver's experience is unique. There are, however, certain general issues that most family caregivers must face, within which every case is different. These general issues can be roughly divided into four categories: memory and judgment problems, behavioral symptoms, changes in ability to carry out day-to-day activities, and medical symptoms and problems. In the next few paragraphs we briefly discuss each of these issues.

Memory and judgment problems. Often these problems are subtle at first: missing a payment on a bill; forgetting a grandchild's birthday; making a purchase that is out of character. Typically the spouse or an adult child will notice these problems and gradually take over more of the decisions, which often goes smoothly. Sometimes, however, a dementia-related judgment error can have catastrophic consequences, such as spending a large portion of one's life savings or having a serious auto accident. As the illness progresses, memory problems affect more and more daily activities—not remembering where the keys were put; accusing someone else of having hidden them; asking the same question over and over. At this stage—when the person can still converse but in a confusing, often disorganized way—caregivers can be especially stressed. Eventually, if the disease goes on long enough, the person may forget or not recognize close family members, including children, grandchildren, or the spouse. Much of this book deals with memory-related issues, including the sections on behavioral symptoms, working with the health care system, and medication management.

Behavioral symptoms. Another category that is often used in describing the effects of dementia is behavioral symptoms. Indeed, many experts say that Alzheimer's disease and other dementias are behavioral disorders, because it's what people do and say that causes much of the difficulty for caregivers. Some behaviors, such as repeated questions, are clearly memory related. Others—such as agitation, suspiciousness, stubborn refusal, and striking out at well-meaning caregivers—result because the person doesn't understand what is going on and, therefore, reacts out of fear or anxiety. For caregivers, it's often helpful to realize that behavioral symptoms are not intended to antagonize anyone, but occur for a reason; therefore, treatment involves trying to problem solve.

Change in the ability to carry out daily activities. As dementia progresses, the individual will begin to need reminders and later hands-on help with daily activities, such as dressing, bathing, and grooming. Later they may develop balance problems, have trouble walking, and perhaps also begin to have urine accidents. At end stages of the illness, some can no longer feed themselves and some need help changing position so as to prevent bedsores. In helping with these daily activities, family caregivers find themselves providing needed support while trying to encourage as much independence as possible. In striking this balance between independence and assistance, it can be helpful to think of yourself as having a variety of techniques that can be ordered based on the extent to which they take over for lost abilities—from set-up (laying clothes out, for example), to giving verbal reminders (to go to the toilet, for example), to guiding the person to start doing the task (starting to brush teeth, and then allowing the person to take over), to doing the entire task for the person.

This process is illustrated graphically in the figure on this page.

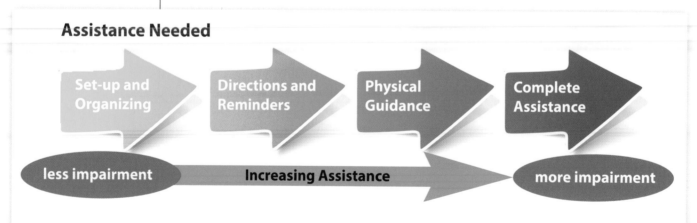

Assistance Needed

Set-up and Organizing → Directions and Reminders → Physical Guidance → Complete Assistance

less impairment → Increasing Assistance → more impairment

Amount of impairment of memory, thinking and self-care capability

In providing assistance with daily activities, such as dressing, the caregiver should provide the amount of assistance that helps get the job done while preserving as much independence as possible.

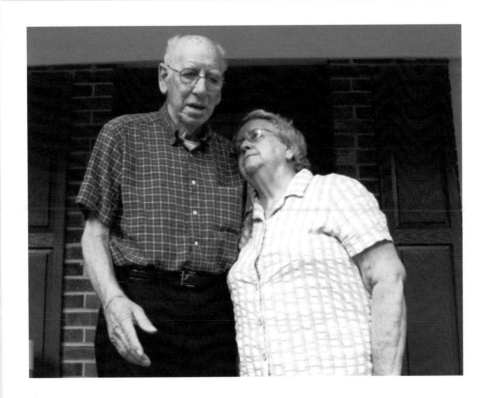

Medical symptoms and problems. The final major category of issues that caregivers must deal with involves all the medical conditions that can occur alongside of or because of dementia. Practically everyone with dementia has other medical problems—hearing trouble, eye problems, arthritis, high blood pressure, diabetes, heart problems, and chronic lung disease are among the most common. The caregiver typically takes over much of the management of these conditions, such as making sure medications are purchased and taken correctly, scheduling doctor's appointments, and monitoring things such as blood pressure and weight.

Particularly challenging for caregivers is knowing what to do when a new problem develops, such as cough or fever, or when an existing problem gets worse; it's challenging in part because the person with dementia may have difficulty explaining what they are feeling, and in part because illness in someone with dementia can express itself in odd ways, such as agitation or refusing to eat. Also, going to the doctor or emergency department is often not a simple matter, because people with dementia may refuse to leave the house, become agitated when away, or have bad events happen because of dementia-related confusion.

A major portion of this book—and indeed a key reason why it has been written—is to help caregivers know what to do when such problems occur. We hope that you find it useful.

> You need to have a caretaker for the caretaker...my sister helped me a lot, even though she's 3,000 miles away.
>
> — *Carol L., caregiver*

> At the end of the day, I write down 3 things that I'm grateful for...just thinking in a positive way helps.
>
> — *Gloria D., caregiver*

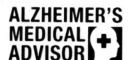

ALZHEIMER'S MEDICAL [+] ADVISOR

Taking Care of Yourself While Helping Someone with Dementia

Even the most well-intentioned, loving family caregivers may be caught off guard by stress-related emotions, fatigue, or illness. Practically every caregiver at one time or another describes feeling "overwhelmed." In addition, the day-to-day personal care required as the illness progresses can lead to physical health problems such as back injuries or infections; so, it's important to take care to protect your own health. What follows is general advice to help you stay well and manage stress during this time of giving care.

Start with You

You need to take care of yourself in order to have something to offer to someone else. Here's how:

Eat Well

Eat a healthy breakfast, lunch and dinner, plus two healthy snacks during the day. Eating in small amounts frequently rather than one or two large meals a day is better for the body and less likely to cause weight gain. Healthy foods include raw fruit; raw, boiled, or steamed vegetables; and grilled or baked meats. Food that is fried is not healthy, and most fast-food restaurant meals are not good either.

In ideal circumstances, caregivers are able to prepare many meals and snacks all at once, called "batch cooking." Make a lot of food at once, freeze in plastic containers, and then thaw as you need it. You can do the same thing with fruits and vegetables you want to use as snacks—wash them, cut them up, and save them in plastic bags or containers.

Part of good nutrition is drinking plenty of fluids. This means six to eight glasses of water a day. Avoid sodas, sweet tea, or other sweet drinks—they add calories and increase your risk of diabetes and heart disease. One or two cups of coffee or tea, and one glass of wine or beer a day is okay if you like them, but drinking more is not healthy.

Get Exercise

This doesn't mean you have to go to a gym, but it does mean you have to be moving. Perhaps you can take a walk together with the person with dementia, if their physical function allows them to join you. If not, see if you can join a friend— it'll help provide motivation and give you someone else to talk with on a regular basis. Aim to get 150 minutes of exercise a week, such as walking or swimming, plus two strength training exercises.

Other examples of exercise are Tai chi, dance, gardening, bowling and yoga which are very low intensity workouts and great at relieving stress. Also, try to get outside when you exercise as fresh air is good for you. By exercising you are increasing your body's natural feel-good hormones which boost your mood and help you relax.

Get Enough Sleep

Sleep is what your body needs to rebuild and repair from a day's activity. For many caregivers, however, getting the recommended minimum of 6 ½ hours a night is difficult, because of having to check on the person with dementia or difficulty sleeping for other reasons. If you can't sleep well at night, you can try catching a catnap when the person you care for naps.

There are certain habits that help you sleep well. These include: going to bed at the same time each night; getting up at the same time each day; making the bedroom quiet and relaxing; having a night light for safety; using your bed only for sleep or sex (not for watching TV or using a computer); and avoiding large meals or exercise for at least two hours before bed time.

Take Time for Yourself

It's common for caregivers to say: "I'm too busy taking care of others to take care of myself." This is understandable, but it's also bad for your health and the care you provide. Instead of toughing it out, ask family or friends to provide care while you give yourself the time you need.

One helpful option is respite care, which offers a break for family caregivers by having paid professionals temporarily provide care. Respite can be provided in the home, in a non-residential community setting, or in a long-term care setting. In-home respite, sometimes called home-care or companion care, involves volunteer or paid help coming into the home on a regular or occasional basis. Community-based respite most often takes place in an adult day center. Residential-based respite, also known as overnight or residential care, provides coverage for a night, a weekend or even a few weeks at an assisted living community or skilled nursing home.

Respite services can refresh the caregiver by providing time to take care of personal issues such as exercising, going to the hairdresser or doctor, shopping, getting together with friends or family, pursuing hobbies, taking a vacation, or just relaxing. Ideally, adequate respite care is in place before the caregiver becomes exhausted or overwhelmed.

Paying for respite care can be a challenge, and funding sources are fragmented. Most health insurance does not cover respite. Potential sources of funds for respite care include Medicare hospice programs, state or veterans' programs, some long-term care insurance programs, and grants from private or non-profit organizations. Read the "Ask for Help" section of this chapter for suggestions.

Be Organized

Getting organized will save a lot of stress in the long run. The sooner this is completed the better. There are two parts: Organizing your own life, and helping organize key issues for the person with dementia.

Organizing your own life is crucial. Here are some tips:

- Get a "calendar" on your phone or buy a calendar/planner. Use it to keep track of your appointments as well as those of the person you're caring for. Also, schedule to clear your refrigerator of old food and check expiration dates on all medicines once a month.

- Have a "family information center" so that others who help in care know what's going on. A bulletin board can be placed in the kitchen, or you can use an online method such as Google calendar.

- Contact your bank to find out what type of support they can provide you for financial management. This will help you pay your bills on time, plan a budget and figure your overall financial picture.

- Sort your mail as soon as you get it. Throw out right away the letters you don't need, and have a place to put things (like bills) that you want to deal with later.

- Invest in a pill organizer for yourself and the person with dementia. Label clearly which is for whom.

- Compile a medical information file for yourself and for the person with dementia. Include an updated list of medications, medical conditions and emergency contact information (see form in Chapter 9). Also include any legal documents you have such as a DNR, living will, or health care power of attorney. Make copies of all the documents; give one to a trusted family member and put another in a place you can get to easily.

- Prepare an emergency kit for your home, in case of a power outage, snowstorm, or other disaster. Items that are especially useful include one or more flashlights, extra batteries, candles and matches, several gallon bottles of water, duct tape, extra blankets, and rain gear.

- In the event something happens to you, it's a good idea to keep a short journal describing the needs, favorite foods, likes and dislikes, and other idiosyncrasies unique to the person you care for.

- Make sure key legal and financial documents are in order and in a safe place. These may include a marriage certificate, divorce papers, military records, a driver's license or other ID, passport, will, living will, durable power of attorney (for financial and health care), insurance policies, and information about safe deposit boxes (number, location, key).

In addition, you'll want to help organize (or take over organizing) for the person with dementia. Even early in the illness this is important, because even early dementia interferes with one's ability to plan and organize well. To the extent possible, involve the person with dementia in this planning. Here are some key things to keep in mind:

- Early in dementia, you'll want to work with an attorney and a health care provider to assure that legal papers are in place in case the person with dementia can no longer make health care decisions. Documents to complete include a **durable power of attorney for health care decisions** (by which people identify whom they'd like to make decisions for them when they are unable), and a **statement of care preferences,** identifying whether and to what extent the person might **not** want certain medical procedures if incapacitated (or dying).

- Early in dementia it's also important to address financial issues. The person with dementia may want to continue to be involved, but some oversight by a family member who reviews bills and payments at least monthly is needed, and usually quite early in the illness it's better for others to manage finances. There's a formal mechanism for designating who should manage finances; one document for doing this legally is the **durable power of attorney for financial affairs.**

- As dementia progresses a person with dementia will likely need help with personal activities such as bathing, dressing, eating, using the toilet, housework, managing money, taking medications, shopping for groceries, caring for pets, and preparing and cleaning up after meals. Although family often provide these services, there are professionals available, too, such as home care aides. It's often hard to know all available resources, so find someone in a medical or social service office who can help you work with the system to obtain the help you need. Make these contacts in advance, before a crisis occurs and you need help right away.

- Well over half of persons with dementia eventually have such intense care needs that they need nursing home or assisted living care. There are, however, many programs to help people with dementia stay at home. Use the internet, friends, the person's health care provider, and local social service agencies (or local aging services) to help you if you are facing this decision.

- Everyone eventually dies, so plan for it. Identify a funeral home and whether to use burial or cremation. Pre-plan what will happen, who will do it, and who will attend whatever ceremonies are planned. Doing this early, when possible, helps incorporate the opinion of the person with dementia.

Listen to Your Body and Get Regular Medical Checkups

You have a lot of responsibility on your shoulders when caring for someone with dementia, and at the same time you have to take care of yourself. If you ignore symptoms of sickness, your health will get worse, and you will not be able to help anyone.

Have a regular doctor, see him or her regularly, and let him/her know that you have care responsibilities. Check in regularly with your health care provider about your diabetes, high blood pressure, or other chronic conditions and make sure you are up to date on your vaccinations. Don't ignore new symptoms such as chest pain, stomach pain, back pain, or leg swelling. If any symptom you have is severe or persistent, contact your medical care provider.

Take your medicines on time and always have them refilled. Have your medication organized so it's easy to take and so that you can grab it and go in an emergency—for example, if you have to take the person you care for to the hospital.

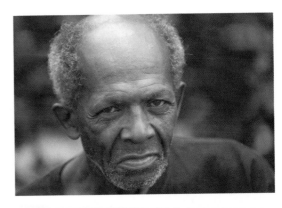

Ask for Help

You can't do everything by yourself, so be willing to ask for help and don't feel bad about it.

For many caregivers, your first source of help is family and friends. Identify who you can trust, and keep in contact with them through regular phone calls. Sometimes families don't know you need help. If you can, talk openly with your brothers, sisters, children, and other family about the help you may need, including financial help and time off from caring.

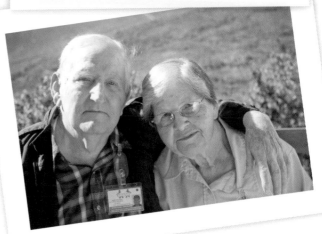

When someone offers to help, have a list ready. Things you might put on that list include shopping, cleaning, car or home repairs, picking up refills, taking the person with dementia out for a few hours (or even days), helping you prepare meals, helping the person with dementia bathe, or staying in with the person while you go out. But, if there's a care task that you especially enjoy doing, ask the person who is helping you to do something else.

Every community has some programs to help caregivers. Often the challenging thing is finding them and getting the help started. If you have internet access, search for "aging services" in your county. Look for your regional Agency on Aging, county aging services, Alzheimer's Association chapter, meals on wheels program, adult day or respite programs, and support groups. Give them a call. If you don't have internet access, use the phone book or ask friends or family to help you with the search. Medical professionals such as doctor's offices can also help you find services that will make your care more manageable.

Attend a support group in person or by phone. These groups can help you express feelings, find help, obtain practical tips on providing care, learn new ways of doing things, and understand that you are not alone or a failure. You may think you are too tired or that you don't need support, but you owe it to yourself to get support.

Keys to Caregiver Wellness

- Eat a healthy diet
- Exercise regularly
- Get enough sleep
- Take time for yourself
- Organize

- Listen to your body
- Get regular medical care
- Be willing to ask for help
- Practice infection prevention

How to Help a Disabled Person Change Position without Injuring Yourself

Many persons with dementia need help changing position, either because of other illnesses (such as stroke, spinal stenosis, or arthritis) or because the disease is in an advanced stage.

If you need to help someone change position, learn and **always** use the techniques that will help prevent you from getting back problems or pulled muscles. Here are the general principles:

- Stand with your feet shoulder width apart.
- Keep the person you are moving close to your body.
- Use your legs and hips to lift, not your back; so, keep your back straight.
- Avoid leaning or stretching.
- Roll or pull the person toward you; never push.
- Tell the person what you are going to do before you do it, and what you want them to do. For example, say "I'm going to help you stand up now. Hold on to my arms and push down with your feet."

How to Sit Someone Up Who Is Lying in Bed

If someone can't sit up from a lying down position
(and you don't have a hospital bed):

1 Position yourself at the side of the bed. Keep your feet shoulder-width apart and knees bent.

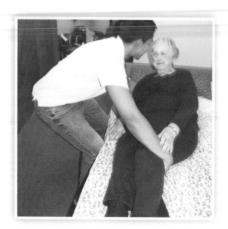

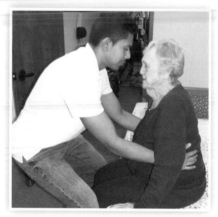

2 Place one of your arms under their legs and the other under their back.

3 Slide their legs over to the edge of the bed while you lift the top part of their body to a sitting position, holding the person close to you because it's better on your back.

How to Help Someone Go From Sitting to Standing

To help someone stand up from a sitting position:

1 Stand in front of them with your feet shoulder-width apart and your knees slightly bent. Do not bend your back.

2 Have the person place their feet flat on the floor, slightly apart.

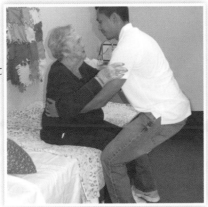

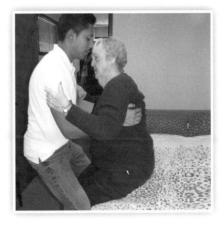

3 Ask the person to place their hands around your arms, while you place your arms around their back and clasp your hands together. If you have a lifting belt, place it around the person's waist and grasp the belt when lifting the person.

4 Lift the person from the seated position, hold them close to you, leaning back slightly and shifting your feet if necessary.

How to Help Someone Sit Down Safely from a Standing Position

As Alzheimer's disease progresses, actions as simple as sitting in a chair can become difficult. When this happens to the person you are caring for, try to guide them to the chair and show them how to sit down. If they still have trouble, or are unsteady on their feet:

1 Position your arms around their trunk while they are standing.

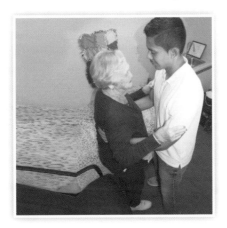

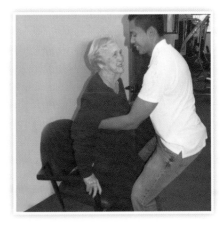

2 Have them place their hands on your upper arms.

3 Pivot or walk them until the back of their knees touches the chair.

4 Then bend your knees and lower the person into the chair. Keep your back straight and do not twist at the waist. If the chair has armrests, have the person place each hand on the corresponding armrest before you lower them, to help with stability.

How to Disinfect Surfaces

- Use a **diluted bleach solution** consisting of ½ cup of bleach in one gallon of water, or a commercially available disinfectant.
- Apply the solution to tables, doorknobs, and other surfaces frequently touched.
- Wearing gloves, wipe the solution onto each surface, allowing it to stay on the surface for at least 5 minutes.
- Then rinse and dry the surface.

Protecting Yourself and Others from Infection

Most common infections are spread from person to person. As a caregiver, your health is very important. Examples of diseases you can contract from or give someone you are caring for are colds, the flu (a respiratory infection), and stomach or intestinal viruses ("stomach flu"). Other than getting adequate rest, good nutrition, staying hydrated and managing your health there are other things you can do to prevent infection.

This is a list of things you should always keep in mind when caring for anyone, whether sick or not.

- Wash your hands in soap and water for 15 seconds before and after helping with personal care such as dressing, bathing, or using the bathroom. Also wash your hands before and after preparing food, eating, or smoking.
- Wear gloves whenever you handle anything that contains spit, vomit, urine, sweat, or bowel material; whenever you touch the person's mouth or a wound; or when you have a cut, sore or rash on your hands.
- You and the person with dementia should stay up-to-date on vaccines, including pneumonia shot, yearly flu vaccine, diphtheria-tetanus shot, and shingles vaccine.

Colds, Sore Throats, Flu, and other Respiratory Infections

All colds, many sore throats, and all flu-like illnesses are caused by a virus and are very contagious. You can catch these illnesses from direct contact with someone who is sick; by breathing the air that has been sneezed or coughed into; or by touching surfaces containing the virus, such as silverware, doorknobs, handles, television remotes, keyboards and telephones.

Here are ways to prevent spreading or getting these illnesses.

Preventing the Spread of Colds, Sore Throats, and other Respiratory Infections

If You Are Sick	If the Person You Care for Is Sick
• Cover your nose and mouth when coughing, sneezing or blowing your nose (to decrease the spread of the virus in the air)	• Avoid touching your eyes, nose, and mouth while providing care
• Wash hands after sneezing	• Wash your hands with soap and water before and after providing care
• Use a hand sanitizer if unable to wash hands	• Have the sick person wear a mask, or wear one yourself
• Wear a mask (available in pharmacies)	• Don't eat or drink from glasses or utensils the sick person has touched
• Stay home and avoid contact with others until 24 hours after your fever is gone	• Get adequate rest and drink plenty of fluids
• Clean and disinfect surfaces and objects that you have touched, using diluted bleach solution or other disinfectant	• Clean and disinfect surfaces and objects that the sick person has touched, using diluted bleach solution or other disinfectant

"Stomach Flu" and Other Infections that Cause Vomiting and Diarrhea

The stomach flu is not a single type of sickness; it can be caused by many different viruses (and on rare occasions, by bacteria). Symptoms are diarrhea, vomiting and cramps. The illness is passed from one person to another through close contact; by sharing food, cups, and eating utensils; or by touching things that have been soiled by the person's spit, vomit, or diarrhea. The viruses that cause this sickness can stay in the person's bowel movements for up to 2 weeks after they feel better, so it's very important to follow precautions to prevent unexpected spread of the illness. Here's what to do:

Preventing the Spread of Stomach Flu and Intestinal Infections

If You Are Sick

- Do not prepare food for others
- Wash hands before eating and after using the bathroom
- Use hand sanitizer if unable to wash hands
- Clean and disinfect surfaces and objects that you have touched, using diluted bleach solution or other disinfectant
- Wear rubber or disposable gloves while handling soiled items, and wash your hands after
- Wash items with detergent at the maximum available cycle length, then machine dry them

If the Person You Care for Is Sick

- Wear gloves when touching soiled clothes or bed sheets, then dispose of gloves after use and wash hands
- Clean and disinfect surfaces and objects that the sick person has touched with diluted bleach solution or other disinfectant
- Wash soiled laundry with detergent at the maximum available cycle length, then machine dry them
- Wash your hands frequently; use hand sanitizer if washing is not convenient

Skin Infections

Skin infections are another condition a caregiver needs to be cautious in taking care of. Symptoms of skin infection are typically a large pimple, a boil, or a red area around a wound or other break in the skin. Infections are typically painful and warm to the touch. Pus or other drainage may be present.

One of the most common skin infections is caused by MRSA (Methicillin-resistant Staphylococcus aureus), a bacterium that is resistant to many antibiotics. This is transmitted by skin-to-skin contact with drainage from a wound, the person's hands (if they've been touching the wound), and bandages or dressings that have been in contact with the wound.

Preventing the Spread of a Skin Infection

- Do not share personal items such as towels, washcloths, razors or clothing
- Keep the wound covered
- Wash hands before and after touching the wound
- Clean and disinfect surfaces and objects that have been in contact with the wound, using diluted bleach or other disinfectant
- Wear rubber or disposable gloves while handling soiled items or wound dressings, and wash your hands after
- Wash items in hot water with detergent at the maximum available cycle length, then machine dry them

> I was able to think back to conversations we had earlier, and it allowed me to honor what he would have wanted. It was a gift and helped me plan confidently.
>
> — *Kathy L., caregiver*

> Get information early, before it feels imminent. The further away from when you'll need it, the better.
>
> — *Gloria D., caregiver*

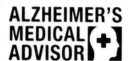

ALZHEIMER'S
MEDICAL [+]
ADVISOR

Setting Goals for Life and Care

People live with dementia. Unfortunately, because dementia is a progressive disease, people also die from and with the disease. Sometimes death is caused by progression of the disease to the point that the body doesn't support normal functions; at other times they die of other long-term or sudden illness, such as heart disease or pneumonia.

It's hard to know the long-range course of dementia. On average people live 8–10 years after diagnosis, but some live shorter and others longer. That's why it's important to set goals for life and care early; such goals can provide guidance throughout the disease process.

Goals of Care

Most simply stated, there are three **goals of medical care**: to prolong life, to maintain function, and to promote comfort (see table below). Typically, prolonging life and maintaining function are the main goals early in the disease, but over time comfort becomes central. Which goal should be prioritized is an individualized decision; it depends on the stage of disease and the person's long-standing preferences. Moreover, at any given time decisions may need to be made between two goals of care. For example, though prolonging life may be important, it may be best to refuse a painful procedure, such as a feeding tube or cancer chemotherapy, if it will cause discomfort and have limited benefit.

Goals of Medical Care and Example Treatment Decisions

Goal	Explanation and Example
Prolong life	Treatment aims to help the person live longer; it could include hospital admission for diagnosis or treatment of new illnesses, use of intravenous medicines and antibiotics (in some cases but not in others), and life support with CPR and a breathing machine
Maintain function	Treatment aims to slow decline and help the person function independently to the extent possible; it could include hospital admission, intravenous medications, physical therapy, and emotional or spiritual care; medical orders may still include preferences to avoid life support or a feeding tube
Promote comfort (palliation)	Treatment aims to improve comfort, maximize quality of life, and preserve capacity for relationships; it may include hospital admission when necessary to improve comfort, medications taken by mouth, hand feeding, hospice services, music, and massage; medical orders will be put in place to not use life support or feeding tubes

Advance Directives

- Another important consideration, related to but different than goals of care, is **advance directives**. Advance directives are legal documents that specify desired care in situations when a person isn't able to make their own medical decisions—they are instructions for care made in *advance*, while the person is still able to make decisions. Types of advance directives vary within states and can address numerous areas; the four most common ones are listed below.

- **Do Not Resuscitate Order (DNR):** Resuscitation means an attempt by medical staff to re-start the heart and breathing in someone whose heart has stopped. A "do not resuscitate" order tells medical personnel **not** to perform resuscitation in those circumstances. A DNR order is important because some state laws do not allow emergency medical workers to obey a living will. It's helpful to discuss the benefits and limitations of cardiopulmonary resuscitation (CPR) with a medical provider in advance of approving a DNR order.

- **Physician (or Medical) Orders for Life Sustaining Treatment (POLST or MOLST):** These are legally binding medical orders that must be followed by doctors and other emergency personnel (including paramedics). They document decisions related to treatment such as for CPR, breathing tubes, feeding tubes, and hospitalization; without them, emergency care staff are required to provide every possible treatment to keep a person alive. The documents have different names in different states, and must be signed by a health care professional. This form should be kept handy and shared when medical care is indicated.

- **Durable Power of Attorney for Health Care (also called a Medical or Health Care Power of Attorney or Health Care Proxy):** This document allows a person to name someone who will make health care decisions if they become unable to do so; it's called "durable" because it remains in effect even after the person being represented becomes unable to speak for themselves. The term "proxy" means that someone has been designated to speak and make decisions for another if that person is unable. Having a durable power of attorney for health care provides a family caregiver with legal authority to make decisions if or when someone with dementia (or other illness) is unable. Obviously, it's important to have discussions about desired health care while an individual is still able to have those discussions, and to document them.

For a person with dementia, assuring that goals of care and advance directives are followed falls to the "proxy"—the close family member or friend who is the **surrogate decision maker** (the person who substitutes for the person with dementia). A durable power of attorney specifies who will serve as the surrogate decision maker. If a power of attorney is not in place, state laws may dictate responsibility for surrogate decision-making to family members or close friends; in this case, the surrogates are not court-appointed and are thus considered informal.

Making Health Decisions When Someone with Dementia is No Longer Able

When serving as a surrogate decision maker, it is helpful to consider two issues: what the person would have wanted, and what is in their best interest.

When thinking about what the person would have wanted, it's helpful to consider the likely outcome of the treatment, any **preferences** the person has expressed about the treatment, the person's religious or personal beliefs, and how the person has felt about similar treatment for someone else. If the surrogate has no information about the person's wishes, then **best interest** comes into play—decisions based on the benefits and burdens of treating and not treating, taking into account the harms and benefits of treatment (including pain and suffering, the degree of potential benefit, and impairment that may result). Surrogate decision-making is not easy, especially if family members disagree on the course of action. It's helpful to know, though, that the law protects surrogates from errors in judgment, and the surrogate is not liable for the consequences of the decision.

At some point, surrogates may be asked whether the time has come for palliative care: providing relief from distressing symptoms and suffering, and improving the quality of time left. Palliative care is provided by specially-trained medical providers who work with a patient's other doctors to provide an extra layer of support. Palliative care is appropriate at **any** stage in a serious illness and can be provided **along with** curative treatment. Hospice is a specific type of palliative care, suitable for people who are considered to be close to death. More information on these options is provided on pages 172–173.

> What is in the person's best interest?

> What would the person have wanted?

> "My husband had bladder cancer before he was diagnosed with dementia. He had his bladder removed and used a bag to collect urine. The bag had to be changed, and after a while he forgot how to close it. I did a lot of laundry.
>
> — *Joan P., caregiver*

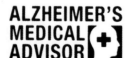

ALZHEIMER'S
MEDICAL [+]
ADVISOR

Common Care Issues

This chapter will help you recognize potential problems, make decisions about what to do, and give you confidence as you provide care.

For each of the medical and behavioral problems in this chapter, you'll find:

- **Basic facts:** This section contains a brief review of the problem, possible causes, and general treatment strategies.

- **Warning signs:** This section has two parts: those signs and symptoms that suggest an emergency; and those that are generally non-urgent but should be brought to a health care provider's attention.

- **Tips on providing relief at home:** In this section, you'll find general tips for providing care at home, and occasionally more specific guidance for particular problems. Often, ways to distract, calm and encourage cooperation with treatment are included.

- **What to watch out for:** When relevant, common complications are listed.

- **Taking care of your own safety and stress:** For certain problems, ways to protect yourself from illness, injury, or stress are discussed.

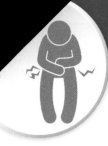

Abdominal Pain

Basic Facts

Abdominal (belly) pain is discomfort anywhere from below the ribs to where the legs begin. Many things can cause belly pain, and in an older person it can be hard to know if it's serious, which is why most people with new belly pain should be seen by a health care provider. Sometimes the symptoms point to a problem that can be taken care of at home, like gas pain, heartburn or constipation. Other times, more serious problems with the liver, gall bladder, pancreas, stomach, intestines, heart or bladder require medical attention.

Signs of a Possible Emergency

Consider calling 911 or taking the person to an emergency department or health care provider office **SOON** if the person has any of these problems:

- **severe pain, or pain that gets worse over time,** especially with **vomiting or fever**
- belly is **swollen, hard** or **very tender** to the touch
- **bloody, black, "tarry", or cranberry colored stool**
- **trouble breathing or shortness of breath**
- **belly pain after a fall or injury**
- **signs of delirium** (see page 48 for more on delirium)
- **vital signs very different from usual,** especially temperature over 100° F (see page 135 for how to measure vital signs)

Other Important Signs

Consider contacting a health care provider by phone and/or setting up a medical visit **within 1–3 days if you notice:**

- **belly pain or diarrhea lasting more than 2 days** (see page 62 for more on diarrhea)
- **belly pain with low grade fever** (see page 70 for more on fever)
- **vomiting lasting more than 24 hours** (see page 130 for more on vomiting)
- **new or worsening constipation** (see page 50 for more on constipation), or **diarrhea after several days of constipation**
- **yellowing of the skin or whites of eyes**
- **weight loss of more than 10 pounds**
- **tiring easily, sleeping more than usual**
- **not eating or drinking well**

What to Watch Out For

- **Severe pain.** A person who has trouble communicating may show severe pain by:
  - writing or seeming unable to get comfortable
  - making sounds like moans, crying or yelling
  - protecting the belly with their arms

See page 141 for more on recognizing pain.

Tips on Providing Relief at Home

As you read this section, keep in mind that belly pain can be a sign of a serious problem. The advice here is not meant to replace the advice of a health care provider.

Here are some problems that can often be managed at home:

▼

Taking Care of Your Own Safety and Stress

When helping someone with diarrhea or similar infections:

- Wash your hands often, and wear rubber gloves when helping with personal care.
- Clean toilet and sink areas well with germ-killing cleaners.

See Chapter 3 for more ways to take care of yourself.

Common Causes of Abdominal Pain: Tips for Caregivers

Problem	Possible clues	What you can try or do
Heartburn, gas, stomach irritation	• Pain after eating, drinking or when lying down after meals • The person frequently takes NSAIDS (pain medications such as ibuprofen or naproxen) or another medicine that can bother the stomach • The person has gas or burping	• Offer smaller meals • Keep the person upright 2-3 hours after meals • Give peppermint or ginger tea • Give 2 tablespoons of a liquid antacid (such as Gaviscon) or two antacid pills (such as Tums) • Avoid chocolate, coffee, alcohol, citrus fruits, NSAID medications
Constipation (see page 50)	• Hard stools • Straining with bowel movements • Bowel movements less often than usual • Person is on a narcotic pain medication	• Offer plenty of fluids and high fiber foods • Try an over-the-counter laxative like Miralax or senna
Blockage in intestines from hard stool	• The person has been constipated for days and then has watery diarrhea	• Don't give medicines for diarrhea • Take the person to a health care provider to have stool taken out
Hemorrhoid or rectal fissure	• Blood on the toilet paper or around the bowel movement • Small amount of bright red blood with bowel movements	• Check the person's anal area for cuts or hemorrhoids • Take them to a health care provider
Stomach virus infection	• Abdominal pain is relieved by vomiting • Sudden vomiting and/or diarrhea • Contact with a sick person 1-4 days before symptoms occur	• Encourage small, frequent sips of fluids, such as Gatorade or soda • Watch for dehydration (page 142) • See information on diarrhea (page 62) or vomiting (page 130)

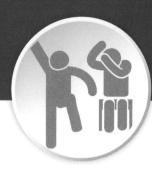

Abuse and Neglect

Basic Facts

Providing care for a person with dementia can be difficult. Most caregivers work hard and do the best they can; however, sometimes there are problems with care. Abuse can be physical (hitting, shoving), emotional (name calling, humiliation, isolation) or sexual (unwanted touching or harassment). Persons with dementia can also become victims of financial abuse, which includes things such as stealing, using dishonesty or fear to get the person to buy something, forging a signature on documents, or cashing checks without permission. Neglect is a failure to meet the person's basic needs for health and safety.

Cases of abuse or neglect that are witnessed or proven should be addressed immediately by moving the person to a safe situation and contacting Adult Protective Services or the police. However, if you're concerned but unsure about abuse or neglect, take time to investigate. These problems can be tricky to clearly identify, as people with dementia can be injury prone, confused about events, and may be uncooperative or unconcerned with personal and home care.

If you're concerned but unsure about abuse or neglect, take time to investigate.

Signs of a Possible Emergency

Consider calling 911 or taking the person to an emergency department or health care provider office **SOON** if the person has any of these problems:

- **serious injury** (such as a broken bone, bleeding that you can't stop)
- signs of **dehydration** (see page 142 for more on dehydration)

Other Important Signs

Consider contacting a health care provider by phone and/or setting up a medical visit **within 1–3 days if you notice these possible signs of abuse and neglect:**

- **unexplained physical injuries** (such as cuts, bruises, or fractures)
- **unexplained bruises, soreness, or bleeding** around the breasts or private areas
- **unexplained weight loss, dehydration, poor hygiene, bedsores** or **unclean living conditions**

Consider taking action yourself, or contacting another family member, attorney, law enforcement or social worker if you notice these possible signs of financial abuse:

- **sudden change in finances** or **unusual purchases**
- the person has **signed legal documents** without knowing their purpose
- **unfamiliar signatures** on checks and other documents, or unexplained changes in the legal will
- previously uninvolved **family members** with a **sudden interest** in the older person
- **unexplained transfer of money** to family members

If you're worried the person is being abused or neglected:

It can be difficult to tell if someone is being abused or neglected. If you notice an unexplained decline in the person's health or behavior, it's worth looking into.

- ☐ Take time to investigate the situation.
- ☐ Gather evidence. Take the person to their health care provider, take photographs, and write down what the potential abuser/neglector says and does.
- ☐ Ask the potential abuser/neglector about your concerns without accusing. For example, you might say: "I've noticed that mother seems to bruise easily. Do you know what happened when she got these?"
- ☐ Talk to the health care provider for advice.

Preventing abuse or neglect:

Providing care for a person with dementia can be overwhelming. Abuse or neglect can happen even when the caregiver has good intentions.

Situations at highest risk for problems include:

- Caregivers with anxiety, depression, drug, alcohol or other mental health problems.
- Caring for a person with many physical needs, or who is uncooperative or aggressive.
- Caregivers who are isolated or without support.

To decrease the chances for physical, sexual or emotional abuse or neglect:

- Consider enrolling the person with dementia in a day program for adults.
- Treat depression, alcoholism, or mental health problems in the caregiver or care recipient.
- Keep the caregiver connected to other people, hobbies, and community support systems.
- Consider professional counseling for the caregiver or for families stressed by caregiving.
- If the person with dementia has an aide or lives in assisted care, check in on them often.
- If the person with dementia has challenging behaviors, talk to their medical provider for advice.

To decrease the chances for financial abuse if the person still manages their money:

- Tell the person not to tell others identifying information (like a bank account number).
- If you notice problems managing money, offer to help. If they refuse and you're concerned, consult an attorney on how to legally take over the finances.
- Put the person on the Do Not Call Registry to reduce contact with telemarketers. Do this by visiting www.DoNotCall.gov or by calling 888-382-1222.
- Watch for large numbers of ads in the mail as the person could be targeted for scams.
- Contact the police if you believe the person has been a victim of a financial scam.

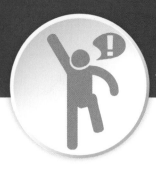

Agitation

Basic Facts

Agitation is a state of being unsettled that can include many behaviors or emotions. A person who's agitated may be grumpy and short-tempered or they may seem worried. They may fidget, ask the same questions over and over again, pace, strike out at something or someone, or yell.

As with other challenging behaviors in persons with dementia, agitation is usually caused by a physical discomfort or need, anxiety, new illness, or situation that's stressful or not stimulating enough. Think of agitation as the person telling you they're overwhelmed and need help. Medicines to treat agitation are usually not as helpful as careful attention to possible causes and then trying different strategies to decrease these triggers.

Signs of a Possible Emergency

Consider calling 911 or taking the person to an emergency department or health care provider office **SOON** if the person has any of these problems:

- **signs of delirium**
  (see page 48 for more on delirium)

- **signs of dehydration**
  (see page 142 for more on dehydration)

- **vital signs very different from usual,**
  especially temperature over 101° F
  (see page 135 for how to measure vital signs)

Other Important Signs

Consider contacting a health care provider by phone and/or setting up a medical visit **within 1–3 days if you notice:**

- **agitation with signs that the person may be getting sick** (like fever, cough, or diarrhea)

- **agitation along with other sudden behavior changes** (like change in their ability to care for themselves, new weakness or sleepiness)

- **new or worsening agitation** lasting more than a day

- the person is **hurting themselves with their fidgeting** (like picking or scratching)

If the person might hurt themselves or others:

- Try to stay calm and reassuring.

- Remove or lock away any unsafe items (guns, knives, heavy objects).

- Try the strategies listed on the next page.

- If you can't calm the person and it's safe to do so, try giving them space. Unless they're in immediate danger, restraining them can make their agitation worse.

- Get help if you need it.

Tips on Providing Relief at Home

A person with new or worsening agitation should be watched carefully for signs of new illness, pain or a physical need. If these are not the cause, problem solve by thinking about the person's situation or routine.

If the person is bored or lonely:

- Distract the person with activities they enjoy. Try calming music, singing, photo sorting, or folding clothes. If possible, take them for a walk or encourage movement in some other way.

- Offer physical touch, like a hug or holding hands.

- For persons with advanced dementia, try giving them something soft to hold, or bringing them near a window or fish tank.

If the person is stressed from a situation:

- Offer calm reassurance and stay positive. Showing your frustration, anger, or worry can make the agitation worse.

- Keep the living area calm, quiet, and well lit.

- Keep a routine for sleep, meals and activities. If needed, try adjusting the schedule (for example, doing more physically demanding activities in the morning).

- Avoid activities and places that are too difficult or hurried, or places that are loud or unfamiliar.

- Make sure the person's glasses and hearing aids are on and working properly.

- Limit caffeine and alcohol.

- If the person is stressed during personal care (like bathing), see page 110 on resisting personal care.

If you think the agitation may be caused by depression (see page 58), hallucinations or delusions (see page 74) or a medication side effect, talk with a health care provider.

If the person is unusually agitated:

- Watch for signs that they're getting sick (like cough or fever), in pain or have a physical need (like hunger, cold or wet).

- If the person is still not themselves after 24 hours, consider contacting the health care provider.

Tip: Keep a routine for sleep, meals and activities. If needed, try adjusting the schedule.

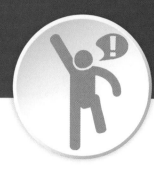

Anger and Aggression

Basic Facts

Nearly half of all persons with dementia will express anger and aggression, whether it's physical (hitting, kicking, destroying things) or verbal (yelling, name-calling, cursing). Sometimes, the behavior is a sign of physical illness or discomfort (body pain, getting a virus, needing the bathroom). Other times, something around them is making them feel stressed or afraid.

No matter what the cause, remember they're not acting this way on purpose. Instead, they're overwhelmed by body sensations or the situation, and they have no other way to express themselves. And although it may be tempting to try a medicine to calm the person down, medicines can cause side effects and usually don't help as much as other strategies. The tips on this page will help you figure out what the triggers are, end an angry or aggressive situation safely, and reduce or prevent problems in the future.

Signs of a Possible Emergency

Consider calling 911 or taking the person to an emergency department or health care provider office **SOON** if the person has any of these problems:

- you're worried the person may hurt themselves or others

- signs of delirium
  (see page 48 for more on delirium)

- signs of dehydration
  (see page 142 for more on dehydration)

- vital signs very different from usual, especially temperature over 101° F
  (see page 135 for how to measure vital signs)

Other Important Signs

Consider contacting a health care provider by phone and/or setting up a medical visit **within 1–3 days if you notice:**

- anger or aggression with signs that the person may be getting sick
  (like fever, cough, or diarrhea)

- anger or aggression along with other sudden behavior changes (like change in their ability to care for themselves, new weakness or sleepiness)

- new or worsening anger or aggression lasting more than a day

If the person might hurt themselves or others:

- Try to stay calm and reassuring.

- Remove or lock away any unsafe items (guns, knives, heavy items).

- Try the strategies listed on the next page.

- If you can't calm them and it's safe to do so, try giving them space. Unless they're in immediate danger, restraining them can make their anger worse.

- Get help if you need it.

Tips on Providing Relief at Home

A person with new or worsening anger or aggression should be watched carefully for signs of new illness, pain or a physical need. If these are not the cause, problem solve by thinking about the person's situation or routine. Think about what happened right before the person became aggressive.

Once you have an idea what may be causing the symptoms, try different strategies until you find what works.

If the person is stressed from a situation:

- Offer your calm reassurance and stay positive. Showing your frustration, anger, or worry can make things worse. You might say: "I'm sorry you're upset. You're safe here."

- If the person is reacting to something you're doing or saying, stop and give them space.

- Distract the person with activities they enjoy. Try calming music, singing, photo sorting, or folding clothes. If possible, take them for a walk or encourage movement.

- Keep the living area calm, quiet, and well lit.

- Maintain a routine for sleep, meals and activities. If needed, try adjusting the schedule (for example, doing more physically demanding activities in the morning).

- Avoid activities and places that make anger worse. These may be activities that are too hard or rushed, or places that are loud or unfamiliar.

- Make sure the person's glasses and hearing aids are on and working properly.

- Limit caffeine and alcohol.

If you think that anger or aggression may be caused by depression (see page 58), hallucinations or delusions (see page 74) or a medication side effect, talk with a health care provider.

If the person is unusually angry or aggressive:

- Check to see if they're feeling ill, have abnormal vital signs, are in pain, or have a physical need (like hunger, cold or wet).

- If the person is still not themselves after 24 hours, consider contacting the health care provider.

What to Watch Out For

- **Anger or aggression during personal care, such as dressing or bathing.** Common causes include pain, or anxiety due to feeling overwhelmed and/or having their personal space invaded.

  - If the person has pain, be especially gentle. Consider giving pain medicine 1–2 hours before the activity.

  - Break the activity into simple steps and give one or two directions at a time.

  - Go slowly and don't rush the person.

  - Explain what you're going to do before you do it, especially before you touch them.

  - Give them simple choices.

  - If they're still having a hard time, step away. You can try again later.

Taking Care of Your Own Safety and Stress

Consider asking someone nearby, like a neighbor, to be ready to help if you need it.

See Chapter 3 for more ways to take care of yourself.

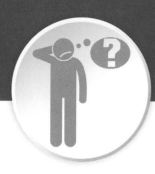

Anxiety or Worry

Basic Facts

We all feel anxious or worried sometimes, but for many persons with dementia, anxiety is a nearly constant part of daily life. Why is this? Partly because at some level the person is aware of what they can no longer do, and in part it's because they often don't understand what is happening around them. In early dementia, common causes of anxiety include worrying about memory loss, changes in relationships with family or friends, and uncertainty about the future. In more advanced dementia, anxiety is often caused by being uncomfortable, not understanding what is going on (including personal care or even normal conversation), or overstimulation from noisy or busy places.

Because the person with dementia often can't say how they feel, their worry comes out in their behavior. They may not want to be around others, become agitated or angry, start wandering or doing things repetitively, or have trouble sleeping. Anxiety can also come along with depression. By figuring out what may be causing the anxiety, you'll be more successful in problem solving.

Signs of a Possible Emergency

Consider calling 911 or taking the person to an emergency department or health care provider office **SOON** if the person has any of these problems:

- **signs of delirium**
  (see page 48 for more on delirium)

- **signs of dehydration**
  (see page 142 for more on dehydration)

- **vital signs very different from usual**, especially temperature over 101° F
  (see page 135 for how to measure vital signs)

Other Important Signs

Consider contacting a health care provider by phone and/or setting up a medical visit **within 1–3 days if you notice:**

- **anxiety with signs that the person may be getting sick** (like fever, cough, or diarrhea)

- **anxiety along with other sudden behavior changes** (like change in their ability to care for themselves, new weakness or sleepiness)

- **new or worsening anxiety** lasting more than a day

If the person might hurt themselves or others:

- Try to stay calm and reassuring.

- Remove or lock away any unsafe items (guns, knives, heavy items).

- Try the strategies listed on the next page.

- If you can't calm them and it's safe to do so, try giving them space. Unless they're in immediate danger, restraining them can make things worse.

- Get help if you need it.

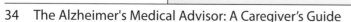

Tips on Providing Relief at Home

A person with new or worsening anxiety should be watched carefully for signs of new illness, pain, or a physical need. If these are not the cause, problem solve by thinking about the person's situation or routine. If the person had anxiety before dementia, think about what sorts of things caused them to worry then. Likely, the same things are troubling to them now.

If the person is stressed from a situation:

- Offer your calm reassurance and stay positive. Showing your frustration, anger, or worry can make things worse.

- Distract them with activities they enjoy. Try calming music, singing, photo sorting, or folding clothes. If possible, take them for a walk or encourage movement.

- Offer physical touch, like a hug or holding hands.

- For persons with advanced dementia, try giving them something soft to hold, or bringing them near a window or fish tank.

- Keep the living area calm, quiet, and well lit.

- Keep a routine for sleep, meals and activities. If needed, try adjusting the schedule (for example, doing more physically demanding activities in the morning).

- Avoid activities and places that make anxiety worse. These may be activities that are too hard or rushed, or places that are loud or unfamiliar.

- Make sure the person's glasses and hearing aids are on and working properly.

- Limit caffeine and alcohol.

If the person is anxious about being forgetful:

- Tell them that you understand how they feel. You might say: "I know this is hard."

- Reassure them that you're here to help.

- Try using humor, by pointing out times that you yourself are forgetful.

If you think the anxiety may be caused by hallucinations or delusions (see page 74) or a medication side effect, talk with a health care provider.

If the person is unusually anxious:

- Check to see if they're feeling ill, have abnormal vital signs, are in pain, or have a physical need (like hunger, cold or wet).

- If the person is still not themselves after 24 hours, consider contacting the health care provider.

What to Watch Out For

See the following pages for more on how to manage behaviors that often come along with anxiety, including agitation (page 30), anger (page 32), depression (page 58), and wandering (page 132).

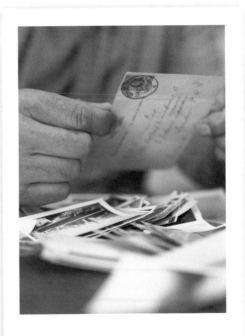

Tip: An activity can often reduce anxious behavior.

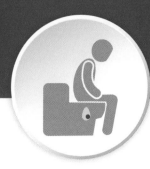

Blood in the Urine

Basic Facts

Blood in the urine can range from harmless to very serious. If the bleeding comes with painful urination, lower back or belly pain, or fever, the person may have an infection. A kidney stone or prostate problem can also cause painful bleeding. On the other hand, painless bleeding can be a side effect of blood thinning medication, or a warning about possible cancer.

Keep in mind that certain medications (like rifampin and pyridium) and foods (like beets, blackberries and rhubarb) can turn urine (or stool) red or orange, giving you a temporary scare.

In any case, if the person you care for has blood in their urine repeatedly, even without other symptoms, they should see their provider.

Signs of a Possible Emergency

Consider calling 911 or taking the person to an emergency department or health care provider office **SOON** if the person has **blood in their urine AND** any of these problems:

- **shaking chills**
- **severe lower belly or back pain**
- an **injury** resulting in blood in the urine
- **blood clots** in the urine
- the person **can't urinate** (except for small amounts), despite feeling like they have to
- the person **pulled out a bladder catheter**
- **signs of delirium**
  (see page 48 for more on delirium)
- **vital signs very different from usual,** especially temperature above 101° F
  (see page 135 for how to measure vital signs)

Other Important Signs

Consider contacting a health care provider by phone and/or setting up a medical visit **within 1–3 days** if the person has **blood in their urine AND:**

- fever above 99° F or 1.2° F above the person's normal body temperature (see page 70 for more on fever) and/or **lower belly or lower back pain** or **painful urination**
- a recent cough, sore throat, cold, or flu
- new swelling in the legs or feet
- repeated episodes of blood in the urine
- sudden changes in urinary habits (new or worse urine accidents, going to the bathroom more often) **lasting for more than 4 days**

If the person pulled out a catheter:

Get medical help right away by having a medical provider come to you or by going to a provider's office or emergency department. **Call 911** if you can't get the person out of the house yourself.

While you wait:

- Stay calm and reassuring. The person is likely in pain.
- Don't try to put the catheter back in.
- If there is bleeding, place clean gauze or a towel over the area. Try to distract the person from the bleeding.

Tips on Providing Relief at Home

Blood in the urine can be scary for someone with dementia. If they're upset by the sight of blood, reassure them that it's not an emergency and that you'll help. If they're also in pain or having other problems, here are some things to try:

If the person has pain with urination, or lower belly/lower back pain:

- Offer at least 6 cups of fluid each day.
- Offer acetaminophen (Tylenol) or another pain reliever recommended by a health care provider.
- Apply a heating pad to the painful area.

If the person has trouble "going"/urinating (urine retention):

- Give privacy and plenty of time in the bathroom.
- Turn on the faucet, place the person's hands in warm water, or run warm water over the private area while they try to urinate.
- Encourage them to lean forward and/or gently push on their belly while on the toilet.
- Get medical help right away if they've gotten little or no urine out after 8 hours, especially if they also have worsening lower belly pain.

If the person is rubbing or scratching their genital area:

- Look for areas of rash or skin problems. If the problem is mild, try an over-the-counter treatment like hydrocortisone cream, A&D ointment, zinc oxide paste, or Vaseline. Otherwise, see a health care provider.
- Gently remind them to not touch the area, and give them something else to do with their hands. See page 30 for tips on agitation.

If the person has a bladder catheter:

- Offer at least 6 cups of fluid each day to keep the bladder flushed out.
- Make sure there aren't kinks in the tubing.
- If the person pulls at the catheter, keep the catheter out of sight by covering it with clothing. Offer a distraction.

What to Watch Out For

- **Urinary Tract Infection:** Blood in the urine can be a sign of a bladder or kidney infection. (See page 124) Tell a health care provider if you also notice these signs:

  - Fever
  - Painful urination
  - Pain in the lower belly or back (Press down on the lower belly and tap the lower back to check for this.)
  - Changes in behavior or more confusion
  - Changes in urinary habits (new or more accidents, going more often)

Taking Care of Your Own Safety and Stress

For your protection, wear disposable gloves when helping with personal care.

See Chapter 3 for more ways to take care of yourself.

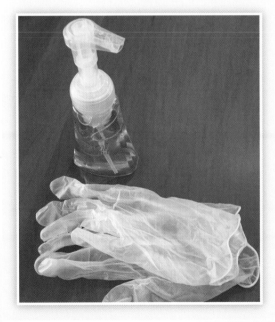

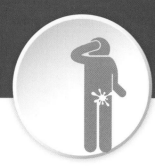

Bowel Incontinence

Basic Facts

Bowel incontinence is when a person leaks stool or has an entire bowel movement by accident. Common causes include not being able to get to the bathroom in time, not recognizing the urge to go, and losing control of the muscles that control bowel movements.

Bowel accidents can be an unavoidable part of advanced dementia. However, if bowel incontinence is new or worsening, check for these treatable causes:

- Side effects of medicines
- Severe constipation
- A chronic bowel disease (such as colitis)
- Diarrhea from an infection or something they ate
- Trouble remembering where the toilet is
- Not staying on the toilet long enough

Bowel incontinence can be very stressful for families and can cause embarrassment or isolation for the person with dementia. After working with a health care provider to identify any treatable causes, try the tips from this guide to make the accidents less frequent and to prevent complications.

Signs of a Possible Emergency

Consider calling 911 or taking the person to an emergency department or health care provider office **SOON** if the person has any of these problems:

- **new or worsening bowel incontinence with diarrhea or fever,** especially if the person has recently been hospitalized on antibiotics
- **bloody, black, "tarry," or cranberry colored stool**
- **severe abdominal pain,** especially with nausea and vomiting
- **vital signs very different from usual,** especially temperature above 101° F (see page 135 for how to measure vital signs)

Other Important Signs

Consider contacting a health care provider by phone and/or setting up a medical visit **within 1–3 days if you notice:**

- **new or worsening bowel incontinence,** especially if accompanied by:
  - **a low-grade fever** for longer than 48 hours (see page 70 for more on fever)
  - **diarrhea and abdominal pain or nausea** lasting more than 2 days
  - **a new medication**
- **more than 6 unformed or watery stools in a 24 hour period** (see page 62 for more on diarrhea)
- **constipation for several days, then bowel incontinence** (see page 50 for more on constipation)
- **greasy, pale, and/or foul smelling stools**
- **red, raw, or open skin** on the buttocks or around the private areas

Tips on Providing Relief at Home

To minimize or prevent bowel accidents:

- Keep access to the bathroom easy by clearing the path of hazards, leaving the door open, or even marking the doorway with bright tape.

- Once in the bathroom, give the person privacy and plenty of time. If they're restless, try playing relaxing music or a giving them a soft object to hold.

- Encourage the use of clothing with Velcro or elastic waistbands.

- If needed, offer simple, step by step instructions and help with wiping, flushing and dressing.

- Note patterns with bowel or bladder accidents and then create a routine. For example, if the person often has a bowel movement after meals, help them to the toilet at this time each day.

- Watch for clues in body language or behavior that the person may need to use the bathroom. For example, they may suddenly pace, begin making sounds, or tug at their clothing. Other times, they may suddenly get quiet or stop what they're doing.

- Prevent constipation with a healthy diet, plenty of fluids, and daily physical activity. See page 50 for more on constipation.

If the person has a bowel accident:

- Try to stay calm and reassuring. If the person seems upset, try a distraction like calming music while you help clean up.

- Take off the soiled diapers or clothing as soon as possible.

- Wash the person's private areas using a soft washcloth, warm water and a mild soap, or adult wipes without fragrance or alcohol. Pat the skin dry before helping them get dressed again.

- If accidents are frequent, apply a moisture barrier such as Vaseline, A&D, or Desitin to protect the skin from irritation.

What to Watch Out For

- **Low fluid in the body (dehydration):** If the person isn't eating or drinking well because they're fearful of having accidents, they may get dehydrated.

  - See page 142 for more on dehydration.

- **Skin rash or infection:** Accidents make skin irritation more likely.

  - Use the tips on this page to keep skin clean and dry.

  - Bring the person to a health care provider if raw or open skin areas develop.

- **Sudden watery diarrhea accidents after being constipated:** The person may have a hard ball of stool (called a "fecal impaction") with watery stool leaking around it.

  - Don't give medicine to stop the diarrhea.

  - Bring the person to a health care provider.

Taking Care of Your Own Safety and Stress

Wash your hands often and wear disposable gloves when helping with personal care.

See Chapter 3 for more ways to take care of yourself.

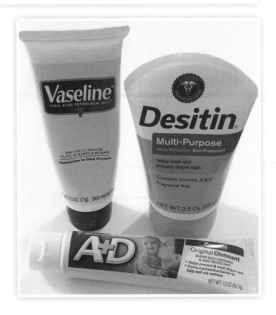

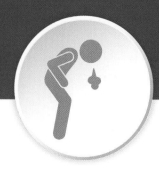

Breathing Problems

Basic Facts

A person who is having trouble breathing might describe feeling winded, short of breath, tightness in the chest, not able to take a deep breath, or unable to get enough air. The problem is often caused by a chronic heart or lung problem, such as asthma, COPD (chronic obstructive pulmonary disease), or heart failure. However, new or worsening breathing difficulty can be a sign of something urgent, like a lung infection, a blood clot in the lungs, a heart attack or allergic reaction. Extreme worry, anger or pain can also cause trouble breathing.

In most cases, a health care provider should be seen for any new or worsening breathing problem.

Signs of a Possible Emergency

Consider calling 911 or taking the person to an emergency department or health care provider office **SOON** if the person has any of these problems:

- **new or worsening trouble breathing while at rest**
- **sudden trouble breathing with any of the following:**
  - **chest pain**, especially if the chest pain started before the breathing problems
  - **chest pain along with leg pain and/or swelling**
  - **rash, itching, and/or swelling**
- **severe shortness of breath**. Here are some signs that the problem is severe:
  - Can't say more than a few words without needing to take a breath
  - Can't lie flat
  - Straining neck muscles to breathe
  - Skin, lips, or fingernails turning purple or blue
- **signs of delirium** (see page 48 for more on delirium)
- **vital signs very different from usual**, especially temperature above 100° F (see page 135 for how to measure vital signs)

Other Important Signs

Consider contacting a health care provider by phone and/or setting up a medical visit **within 1–3 days if you notice:**

- **new or worsening trouble breathing when active** (such as climbing the stairs)
- **trouble breathing when the person is worried, angry, or has pain**

Tips on Providing Relief at Home

Here are some things you can try at home to bring short-term relief for breathing problems. Remember to visit a health care provider to find the cause of the breathing problem and follow any instructions for your situation.

- Help the person into an easier-breathing position, such as:
  - Sitting, leaning forward with elbows to the knees.
  - Standing, leaning against a wall with hands to thighs.
  - In bed, sitting upright using pillows.
- Help the person relax with slow, deep breathing techniques. These work best if the person can follow directions and has practiced beforehand. Say something like this:
  - "Breathe in through your nose. When you breathe out, breath slowly and purse your lips like you're whistling."
  - "Put your hand on your belly. Breathe so it makes your hand rise and fall with each breath."
- Try playing calm, slow music.
- Try blowing cool air gently on their face.
- Try distracting them with something they enjoy doing.
- Give them space if needed.
- If the person has asthma:
  - Avoid triggers like smoke or pets.
  - Use medicines as directed.
- If the person gets short of breath during everyday activities, like showering or getting dressed:
  - Take breaks often.
  - Put chairs in places around the house for rest. Use a shower seat.
  - Offer a healthy, high fiber diet with smaller meals throughout the day. Encourage calm, quiet activities in the hour after eating.
  - Ask the health care provider if an exercise program might help.
- If you think the breathing problems are due to worry or anger, see pages on anxiety, agitation and anger in this book.

If the person has sudden, severe trouble breathing:

- In most cases **call 911**.
- Things you can do right away:
  - Try to stay calm and reassuring.
  - If they have asthma, give them a dose of their fast-acting inhaler.
  - If they're having an allergic reaction and they have an Epi-pen, give it. Otherwise give diphenhydramine (Benadryl).
  - If they're choking, do back blows and belly thrusts. (See page 46)

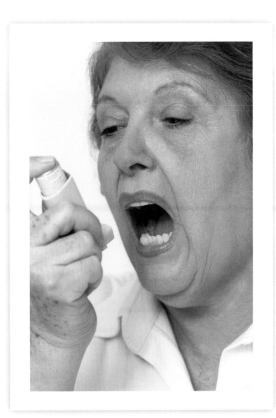

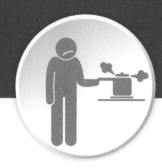

Burns

Basic Facts

A person with dementia is often less able to judge safety around the home, putting them at risk of burn injuries. Common causes of burns include sun exposure, hot bath or shower water, food or drink (like hot tea, noodles, or potatoes), electricity, chemicals, and a hot object such as a stove, fireplace or curling iron. Breathing in smoke or steam can cause burns in the mouth, throat and lungs.

The severity of the burn and how it's treated depend on where the burn is, how large it is, and how deep it goes. Minor burns affecting only the top layer of skin are called **first-degree burns**. These will cause skin redness and mild swelling without any blistering, and take about a week to heal. If the burn affects both the top layer of skin and the tissue underneath, it's a **second-degree burn**. These burns form fluid-filled blisters and can take 3 or more weeks to heal. The most serious and deep burn is a **third-degree burn**. These may look white, brown or charred from burned muscle, fat and nerves. Third degree burns can take months to heal and may require skin grafting.

Signs of a Possible Emergency

Consider calling 911 or taking the person to an emergency department or health care provider office **SOON** if the person has any of these problems:

- **large or deep burns involving the face or hands**
- **trouble breathing, shortness of breath or coughing,** especially after breathing in smoke or steam
- **passing out** (even if only for a few seconds)
- **shaking chills**
- **temperature above 101° F** (see page 135 for how to measure vital signs)

Other Important Signs

Consider contacting a health care provider by phone and/or setting up a medical visit **within 1–3 days if you notice:**

- any burn that is more than a couple of inches wide; looks white, brown or charred in color; or has blisters in more than one place
- signs of infection in a burn:
  - increasing redness, pain, swelling or warmth around the burn
  - increased leaking of fluid (especially pus) from the burn
- signs that the person may be abused or neglected (see page 28 for more on abuse and neglect)

Tips on Providing Relief at Home

To treat a minor burn at home:

- After running under cold water, clean the area with a mild soap and saline or water.
- If the skin is broken or a blister has formed and popped, apply a moisturizer such as Vaseline. Try not to pop blisters as these help protect the wound.
- Cover the wound with a non-stick bandage like Telfa. Try to avoid putting tape directly on the skin; instead, wrap the area with gauze from a roll or use an Ace bandage.
- For temporary pain relief, use acetaminophen (Tylenol) or another pain medication recommended by their health care provider.
- Aloe vera may also help soothe pain from a minor burn, but will not help with healing.
- Make sure the person is up-to-date on their tetanus shot.

To help prevent cooking and food related burns:

- Help the person with cooking.
- Check food and drink to be sure they've cooled before serving.
- Avoid loose fitting clothes when cooking, as they may catch fire more easily.
- Keep a fire extinguisher in the kitchen.

Other home safety tips:

- Set the hot water temperature to no more than 120° F (49° C).
- Check smoke alarm batteries regularly.
- Be careful when using candles, a space heater, or curling iron.
- If someone in the home smokes:
  - Use electronic cigarettes or smoke outside. Never smoke in bed.
  - Keep cigarettes, lighters, matches, and other smoking materials in a safe place.
  - Place a deep, sturdy ashtray away from anything that can burn.
  - Don't throw cigarettes into mulch, potted plants, landscaping, peat moss, dried grasses, or leaves.
  - Before you throw away butts and ashes, make sure they're completely extinguished.
  - Never smoke where medical oxygen is used.

If the person has just been burned:

- Try to stay calm and reassuring.
- For safety, put out any fire, turn off electricity or put on gloves before touching chemicals.
- Remove the person from the heat or chemical. If needed, take clothes or jewelry off. Avoid removing items stuck to the skin.
- Run cool water over the area for 10–15 minutes or until the pain eases. Use a large amount of water to remove chemicals.
- If the burn seems large or deep, or if the person is having trouble breathing, consider calling 911.
- If the burn seems minor, see the tips on this page.
- If you're unsure about the seriousness of the burn, wrap the area in a clean cloth and bring the person to a health care provider.

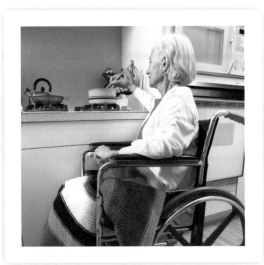

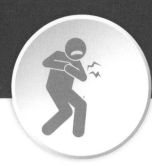

Chest Pain

Basic Facts

It can be frightening when a person has chest pain and you're not sure of the reason, especially if the person can't communicate well. The truth is, even health care providers can have a hard time knowing how serious the problem is over the phone. So, even though the cause may be as simple as gas, providers will generally advise that the person be brought to an emergency department (ED) to be checked carefully.

When deciding what to do about chest pain, think about the situation. Has the person had this type of pain before, and it ended up to be not serious? If so, you may know what to try at home first to bring relief. Remember to consider the person's care plan. If the person has "DNR" orders, or if bringing them to the ED in the past has caused a lot of problems, you may think twice before calling 911.

This guide can help you with these hard decisions. What to do won't always be easy or obvious. Do what feels right and try to accept what comes without second guessing yourself.

Signs of a Possible Emergency

Consider calling 911 or taking the person to an emergency department or health care provider office **SOON** if the person has any of these problems:

- **passing out** (even if only for a few seconds)
- **trouble breathing or shortness of breath**
- pain worrisome for heart attack: **squeezing or heaviness in center of chest, pain going to the left arm, shoulder or jaw**
- **pain similar to a previous heart attack**
- **pain that doesn't stop,** especially if it keeps getting worse
- **sweating, nausea, or vomiting with pain**
- **vital signs very different from usual** (see page 135 for how to measure vital signs)

If the person has a chest pain emergency:

If the person has any warning signs of emergency (see panel to the right), **try to stay calm and, in most cases, call 911.** While you're waiting:

If the person is awake:
- Help them get as comfortable as possible.
- Try lying them down with head propped.

If the person is passed out:
- Check if the person is breathing or has a pulse.
- If there is no breathing or no pulse, and resuscitation is part of the care plan, start CPR (cardiopulmonary resuscitation). To learn CPR, call the American Heart Association at 1-877-242-4277 or visit www.cpr.heart.org.
- If they're breathing and have a pulse:
  - lie them on their side to prevent choking
  - loosen tight clothes
  - cover them with a blanket if it's cold

Other Important Signs

Consider contacting a health care provider by phone and/or setting up a medical visit **within 1–3 days if you notice:**

- **pain that gets better with rest but comes back with exercise**
- **pain that doesn't get any better after home treatment**
- **pain that appears severe in a person whose care plan includes not going to the hospital**

Tips on Providing Relief at Home

Chest pain can always be a sign of a life-threatening problem, such as a heart attack or blood clot in the lungs, even if the person doesn't look bad. Use this information, along with the advice of your health care provider, to help you make decisions and provide relief.

As with any pain, get the person into a comfortable position in a chair or bed. While you're deciding what to do, try distraction with calming music or a favorite TV show.

This table gives tips for chest pain caused by less serious problems.

Taking Care of Your Own Safety and Stress

Making hard health care decisions can be stressful. To lessen your stress:

- Know the person's medical care wishes and have a written care plan to guide you. (See Chapter 4)

- Talk with family members and try to get everyone on the same page before emergencies.

- Talk to a trusted health care provider about your options.

See Chapter 3 for more ways to take care of yourself.

Common Causes of Chest Pain: Tips for Caregivers

Problem	Possible clues	What you can try or do
Heartburn, gas, or stomach irritation	• Pain after eating, drinking or when lying down after meals • Gas or burping • Use of NSAIDS (such as ibuprofen or naproxen) or another medicine that can bother the stomach • The person has had heartburn before, and this is similar	• Smaller meals • Stay upright 2-3 hours after meals • Peppermint or ginger tea • 2 tablespoons of a liquid antacid (such as Gaviscon) or two antacid pills (such as Tums) • Avoid chocolate, coffee, alcohol, citrus, and NSAIDS such as ibuprofen (Advil) or naproxen (Aleve)
Bone or muscle pain	• Pain is sharp, or like a pinprick (NOT "squeezing" or "heavy") • Pain is worse with a deep breath or twisting, and the person's vital signs are normal • Pain was clearly brought on by coughing or physical straining (like lifting something) • There's a place on the chest tender to the touch	• Pain medicine like Acetaminophen (Tylenol) (talk to a health care provider about dose or restrictions) • Position the person so that they're most comfortable (it may help to lie on the side that hurts, or on the other side) • Place an ice pack or heating pad on the area that hurts (wrapped in a towel to protect the skin)

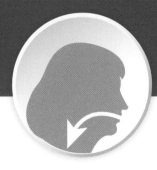

Chewing and Swallowing

Basic Facts

Problems with chewing and swallowing can make mealtimes stressful. You might find the person with dementia eats very slowly or needs reminders to chew and swallow. They also may have trouble getting their mouth and throat muscles to work together, causing them to cough or choke, or to "pocket" food in their cheeks. Over time, the person may lose weight or get dehydrated.

If after reading this guide you're worried about the person's chewing and swallowing, consult their health care provider. If you want more advice, specialists like geriatricians or speech therapists and ear, nose and throat doctors may help.

If the person chokes on food:

If the person chokes and isn't making any noise (not coughing or talking):

- This means they can't get air in or out.
- Stay with the person and try to stay calm.
- Have someone call 911.
- Give 5 back blows:
  With the heel of your hand, give 5 hard blows between the person's shoulder blades.
- If still choking, give 5 belly thrusts (Heimlich maneuver):
  - Standing behind the person, wrap your hands around their waist.
  - Place your fist under their ribs, with your other hand on top.
  - Give 5 quick thrusts up.
- If the person passes out:
  - Start CPR (cardiopulmonary resuscitation). To learn CPR, call the American Heart Association at 1-877-242-4277 or visit www.cpr.heart.org.

If the person chokes and is scared but *can* make noise or cough:

- This means they can get air in and out.
- Stay calm and tell the person to cough if they can.
- If they're not getting better, do back blows and belly thrusts (see above) and call 911.

Signs of a Possible Emergency

Consider calling 911 or taking the person to an emergency department or health care provider office **SOON** if the person has any of these problems:

- **if the person chokes, struggles to breathe or passes out** (see panel on left)

Other Important Signs

Consider contacting a health care provider by phone and/or setting up a medical visit **within 1–3 days if you notice:**

- **sudden severe coughing, voice changes or noisy or wet-sounding breathing** during or right after eating or drinking (Contact the health care provider within 24 hours.)
- **pain, coughing, choking, drooling or food or liquid coming out of the nose** when eating or drinking
- **food or drink is often spit out, feels "stuck" in throat, or is kept "pocketed" in the mouth instead of swallowing**
- **sleepiness** while eating
- **teary eyes or a running nose** during or after swallowing
- **eating very slowly (longer than 30 minutes)**
- **you're worried the person isn't eating or drinking enough**
- **weight loss of more than 10 pounds over 1–3 months**

Tips on Providing Relief at Home

Here are some things you can try at home when the person has trouble chewing and/or swallowing. Be sure to also visit a health care provider for advice on your situation.

- Offer food when the person is most awake and sitting upright.

- Try offering small meals and snacks throughout the day instead of 3 large meals.

- Make sure mealtime isn't rushed. Keep noises low and TV off, or try playing calm music.

- Always stay close by for safety.

- Try offering a sip of drink after each bite, or, if needed, gently remind them to swallow before the next bite.

- Try changing the foods you offer or how they're prepared. You might try thick milkshakes, pureed fruits or vegetables, moistened bread or meat, food cut into bite-sized pieces, or a sippy cup for drinking. Stay away from sticky, very hot, or very cold foods.

- Help them clean their teeth regularly. See page 56 for dental problems.

- Work with a therapist to learn ways to make eating and drinking safer and easier.

- See page 98 if you're worried the person isn't eating or drinking enough.

What to Watch Out For

- **Choking:** Know what to do in a choking emergency (see page 46) and always stay close by when the person is eating.

- **Lung infection:** Swallowing problems can cause food and drink to get into the lungs. Watch for signs of lung infection, including:

  - Fast breathing, changes in breathing sounds
  - Changes in vital signs, including fever

- **Low fluid in the body (dehydration):** If the person with dementia isn't eating or drinking well, they can quickly become dehydrated. Some signs of dehydration are:

  - Dry mouth and tongue
  - Urinating very little
  - Fast heart beat
  - Slow, weak, or low energy

  If you've tried the tips on this page but the person still seems dehydrated, get medical help.

- **Weight loss:** Weight loss can happen if the person isn't getting enough calories. In addition to the tips on this page:

  - Take the person to the health care provider to be checked, especially if they've lost more than 5 pounds in a week or 10 pounds in 1–3 months.
  - Offer high calorie full-fat foods, like milkshakes. Talk to a nutritionist for ideas.

Taking Care of Your Own Safety and Stress

When helping a person who has chewing and swallowing problems:

- Never put your hand or fingers between their teeth.

- Be prepared in case of a choking emergency.

See Chapter 3 for more ways to take care of yourself.

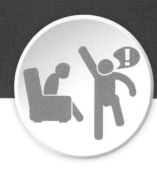

Confusion and Delirium

Basic Facts

A gradual increase in confusion over months to years is common as dementia progresses. Sometimes worsening confusion develops more quickly, over hours to days. When this happens, it's important to pay close attention.

If the confusion seems mild or moderate and happens in the early afternoon or evening, only to get better with a night's rest, it is likely sundowning (see next page). If the timing doesn't seem right for sundowning, think about other possible causes like dehydration (see page 142), a virus, not sleeping well, or a reaction to a new medicine. If the person is having other new symptoms along with worsening confusion, consider taking them to their health care provider.

If the worsening confusion is sudden and severe, it may be delirium (see 'Signs of a Possible Emergency' for a complete list of signs). Delirium is commonly caused by a serious medical illness, medication side effects, or is a complication after surgery. Luckily, once the cause is treated, the person gets back to being himself or herself.

If the person might hurt themselves or others:

- Try to stay calm and reassuring.
- Remove or lock away any unsafe items (guns, knives).
- Try the strategies listed on the next page.
- If you can't calm them and it's safe to do so, try giving them space. Try not to physically hold them back unless you must for safety.
- Get help if you need it.

Signs of a Possible Emergency

Consider calling 911 or taking the person to an emergency department or health care provider office **SOON** if the person has any of these problems:

- **two or more of the following delirium signs:**
  - more than usual trouble paying attention
  - more than usual trouble with memory, thinking or speaking
  - change in energy level (very sleepy or very active)
  - new hallucinations, delusions or strong emotions (crying with sadness, screaming with anger)
  - changes develop quickly (hours to days)
  - changes come and go over the course of the day (for example, sometimes awake and alert, then suddenly hyperactive and confused)
- **vital signs very different from usual,** especially temperature over 101° F (see page 135 for how to measure vital signs)

Other Important Signs

Consider contacting a health care provider by phone and/or setting up a medical visit **within 1–3 days if you notice:**

- **the person has one or two mild delirium signs** (see 'Signs of a possible emergency' above)
- **the person has signs of "sundowning" for the first time** (see page 49 for more on sundowning)

Tips on Providing Relief at Home

If the person you care for has signs of delirium, seek medical care for diagnosis and treatment. While under care, here are some tips:

If the person is confused and upset:

- Offer calm reassurance with kind words and gentle touch. You might say: "I know you're upset. I'm right here. Would it help if I held your hand?"

- Make eye contact and speak in simple, clear sentences.

- When helping with daily activities, remind the person who you are and say what you're about to do. You might say: "I'm your daughter and I'm going to help you out of bed now."

- Try different ways to remind the person of where they are, the time and the day.

  - Keep a clock, calendar, or a board with a daily schedule somewhere visible.

  - Give gentle reminders during conversation. You might say: "I'm so glad that I, your husband, can spend time with you this Sunday morning."

- Keep the area around the person calm and familiar.

  - Try playing calm music, using soft lighting, and keeping the temperature comfortable.

  - As much as possible, have family and other familiar people spend time around the person. However, avoid having too many visitors at one time.

  - Try to stick to a daily routine for sleeping, eating and activities.

- Try distraction with calming activities they enjoy.

- If the person is tired or unusually confused, encourage them to sleep.

- Encourage the person to walk or move. If they're unsteady, stay close by for support.

- Encourage use of eyeglasses or hearing aids, and make sure they're working properly.

- To prevent dehydration, encourage at least 4-6 cups of fluid each day.

If the person with delirium is in the hospital:

- Try to have at least one family member stay at their side at all times until they get better.

- Ask a health care provider if any medical devices (catheters, IV) can be taken out.

What to Watch Out For

- **Behavior changes:** See the following pages for more on how to manage the challenging behaviors possible with delirium: agitation (page 30), anger (page 32), anxiety (page 34), hallucinations/delusions (page 74), and wandering (page 132).

- **Low fluid in the body (dehydration):** Delirium can lead to poor eating and drinking. See page 142 for more on signs of dehydration and how to prevent it.

- **Falls:** Delirium puts the person at higher risk of falling and injuries. See page 68 for more on falls and how to prevent them.

About Sundowning:

"Sundowning" refers to confusion, agitation or restlessness that begins or worsens in the late afternoon or early evening as light begins to fade. Although the causes are not well understood, there are things you can do to help:

- Keep the home well lit, quiet and calm.

- Offer distraction with a calming activity as an evening routine.

- Avoid big meals, alcohol or sweets at night.

- Encourage healthy activity and sleep routines. See pages 116 and 118 for more on sleep.

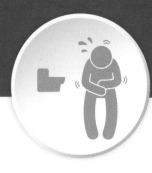

Constipation

Basic Facts

Constipation is when someone has trouble making a bowel movement (pushing out stool) or doesn't have one often enough. Here are some clues the person may be constipated:

- Straining or pushing very hard with bowel movements
- Hard stools
- 2 or fewer bowel movements a week
- Feeling like they still "have to go" after a bowel movement, like there's something blocking stool from coming out, or needing to use fingers to get stool out

Constipation can be uncomfortable, but it's usually not an emergency. Eating a high fiber diet with plenty of fluids, being as physically active as possible, and taking over-the-counter (non-prescription) stool softeners can bring relief. If these tips don't help, talk to the person's health care provider, especially because constipation is sometimes caused by a medication.

Signs of a Possible Emergency

Consider calling 911 or taking the person to an emergency department or health care provider office **SOON** if the person has any of these problems:

- **severe or worsening belly pain,** especially after eating
- **belly is swollen, hard or very tender to the touch**
- **bloody, black, "tarry," or cranberry colored stool**
- **vomiting,** especially if the person hasn't had a bowel movement in a week or more
- **signs of delirium** (see page 48 for more on delirium)
- **vital signs very different from usual,** especially temperature above 101° F (see page 135 for how to measure vital signs)

Other Important Signs

Consider contacting a health care provider by phone and/or setting up a medical visit **within 1–3 days if the person:**

- has several days of no bowel movements, then diarrhea or watery stool
- has belly pain or discomfort
- feels bloated or full
- has constipation that's new or getting worse
- has lost 10 or more pounds over 1–3 months
- tires easily and sleeps more than usual
- has a fever for longer than 48 hours (see page 70 for more on fever)

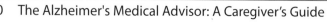

Tips on Providing Relief at Home

To prevent and treat constipation:

- Keep track of how often and when the person has a bowel movement. Learn what's normal for them.

- Offer plenty of fluids. Aim for the person to drink between 4 and 6 cups of their favorite non-alcoholic and non-caffeinated fluid every day.

- Encourage the person to eat a healthy, high fiber diet. Fiber helps keep the digestive tract moving. Fruits, vegetables and whole grains are high in fiber. Aim for between 20–35 grams of fiber every day. Read food labels and pick foods that have high "dietary fiber" per serving.

- If it's hard for the person to get enough fiber from food, try an over-the-counter fiber supplement like psyllium seed (Metamucil), methylcellulose (Citrucel), calcium polycarbophil (Fibercon), or wheat dextran (Benefiber).

- Help the person stay active. Physical activity, even just walking, helps move the bowels.

- Encourage the person to sit on the toilet right after meals. This is when the bowels are most active.

- If the person remains constipated despite these efforts, try a dose or two of an over-the-counter laxative. There are many kinds available, including milk of magnesia, magnesium citrate, bisacodyl (Dulcolax), Miralax, or senna (Senokot). Ask a health care provider before using milk of magnesia or magnesium citrate.

- If you've tried these tips without relief, consult a health care provider.

Taking Care of Your Own Safety and Stress

When helping someone with constipation:

- Wash your hands often and wear rubber gloves when helping with personal care.

- Clean toilet and sink areas well with germ-killing cleaners.

See Chapter 3 for more ways to take care of yourself.

What to Watch Out For

- **Hemorrhoids and anal tears:** Constipation and passing hard stools can cause hemorrhoids (swollen blood vessels around the anus) and anal tears (cuts). These problems can lead to bleeding. If you see bright red blood when wiping the anus or in the toilet bowl:

  - Check the anal area for swelling or cuts.

  - Soak the anal area in shallow, warm water (called a Sitz bath). Ask the pharmacy about a plastic tub that fits over the toilet for easier soaking.

  - Try over-the-counter creams and wipes for hemorrhoids.

- **Sudden watery diarrhea after being constipated:** The person may have a hard ball of stool (called a "fecal impaction") with watery stool leaking around it.

  - Don't give medicine to stop the diarrhea.

  - Bring them to the health care provider who'll remove the hard stool.

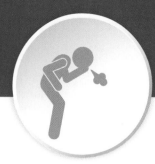

Cough

Basic Facts

Coughing is an important reflex that protects the lungs by helping the body get out any foreign substances, such as food, mucus, or smoke, thereby helping prevent serious injury or infection.

A cough can also, however, be very bothersome. Common causes include:

- Viral infections, including colds, the flu, and bronchitis

- Chronic health problems, such as COPD (chronic obstructive pulmonary disease), asthma, heartburn, heart failure, and allergies

- Certain blood pressure medications, called ACE inhibitors (cough is a common side effect)

Less common but important additional causes of cough include pneumonia or a blood clot in the lungs.

If the person has cough and severe trouble breathing:

In most cases **call 911**. While you're waiting for help:

- Try to stay calm and reassuring.

- If they have asthma, give them a dose of their fast-acting inhaler.

- If they're having an allergic reaction and they have an EpiPen, give it.

- If they're choking, do back blows and belly thrusts. (See page 46)

- See page 40 for more tips on breathing problems.

Signs of a Possible Emergency

Consider calling 911 or taking the person to an emergency department or health care provider office **SOON** if the person has any of these problems:

- **coughing up a large amount of mucus or blood** (more than 1 cup in 24 hours)

- **sudden trouble breathing with any of the following:**

  - **chest pain**, especially if the chest pain started before the breathing problems

  - **both chest and leg pain and/or swelling**

  - **rash, itching, and/or swelling**

- **severe shortness of breath** (see page 40 for more on breathing problems)

- **signs of delirium** (see page 48 for more on delirium)

- **vital signs very different from usual,** especially temperature above 101° F or breathing rate over 25 (see page 135 for how to measure vital signs)

Other Important Signs

Consider contacting a health care provider by phone and/or setting up a medical visit **within 1–3 days if you notice:**

- **cough lasting longer than 10 days** or getting worse over time

- **coughing fits so severe that they cause fainting or vomiting**

- **coughing up small amounts of blood, or pink, rust-colored or red-streaked mucus** (phlegm)

- **coughing up yellow or green mucus** (phlegm)

- **fever, chills, muscle aches, and/or headaches**

- **any trouble breathing or change in other vital signs** (see page 135 for how to measure vital signs)

- **new or worsening swelling in the ankles, feet, or legs**

- **unintentional weight loss**

Tips on Providing Relief at Home

For short-term relief for cough:

- Offer lots of fluids like water, soup, and juice. These can relieve irritation and loosen mucus.

- Use a humidifier, a steam vaporizer, and/or encourage the person to take a steamy shower.

- Try an over-the-counter cough medicine or drops. If you do, follow the label closely and talk with a pharmacist about any interactions with other medications the person takes.

- Avoid cough triggers like cigarette smoke, perfumes, dust and pollen.

- If the cough is causing a sore throat, rib pain, or headache, use acetaminophen (Tylenol) or another pain medication if recommended by the person's health care provider.

- If the person smokes and might be willing to stop, ask a health care provider for help.

If the cough is due to heartburn (acid reflux):

- Limit high fat foods, chocolate, coffee, colas, acidic juices (like orange juice), and alcohol.

- Avoid food or drink for 3 hours before lying down.

- Raise the head of the bed six to eight inches.

If the cough is due to allergies or asthma:

- Avoid triggers (like dust or pollen).

- Try an over-the-counter allergy medicine such as loratadine (Claritin), fexofenadine (Allegra), or cetirizine (Zyrtec). For asthma, take prescription medicines as directed.

What to Watch Out For

In addition to the tips on this page, consider talking with a health care provider if any of these problems develop with the cough:

- **Trouble sleeping:** Cough can keep the person up at night. Try a humidifier by the bed. See the health care provider if the person is having trouble breathing while lying down.

- **Exhaustion:** Frequent coughing uses a lot of energy and can wear the person down.

- **Painful coughing:** This is sometimes due to a pulled muscle or a bruised or broken rib, but it could also be a sign of a more serious problem (such as pneumonia).

- **Urine leakage:** Coughing can cause urine to leak, especially in older women. See page 122 for more on urine leakage.

- **Cough lasting longer than 10 days or getting worse:** This may be a sign that other treatment is needed.

- **Vomiting after severe coughing:** Instead of 3 large meals, offer smaller meals and snacks throughout the day.

Taking Care of Your Own Safety and Stress

If the cough is due to an infection:

- To prevent spread of germs, wash your hands often and, if possible, have the person wear a mask. If they can't wear one, wear one yourself.

- Get your flu shot each year.

- Healthy diet, exercise, and sleep will help you stay healthy.

See Chapter 3 for more ways to take care of yourself.

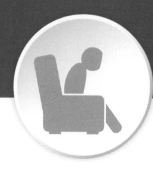

Decreased Activity

Basic Facts

Persons with dementia commonly have periods where they slow down, don't do anything, or seem sleepy or weak. This "slowness" may be caused by physical trouble getting around, pain, medication side effects, depression or feeling overwhelmed by too much activity around them. Dementia can also cause difficulty getting started on an activity. For example, the person may sit and stare at a closed photo album until someone opens it.

While these symptoms can be due to dementia, a sudden and severe change in the person's activity level, especially when it comes along with other changes, deserves your careful attention. It could mean the person has a medication side effect, is dehydrated, or is getting sick.

Signs of a Possible Emergency

Consider calling 911 or taking the person to an emergency department or health care provider office **SOON** if the person has **decreased activity PLUS** any of these problems:

- any possibly urgent medical problem such as **chest pain, trouble breathing, or a sudden change in their ability to move certain parts of their body**

- **signs of delirium** (see page 48 for more on delirium)

- **signs of dehydration** (see page 142 for more on dehydration)

- **vital signs very different from usual,** especially temperature over 101° F (see page 135 for how to measure vital signs)

Other Important Signs

Consider contacting a health care provider by phone and/or setting up a medical visit **within 1–3 days if you notice:**

- **decreased activity with signs that the person may be getting sick** (like fever, cough, or diarrhea)

- **decreased activity along with other sudden behavior changes** (like change in their ability to care for themselves)

- **new or worsening decreased activity, sleepiness or whole body weakness** lasting more than a day

- **unplanned weight loss**

If the person seems slow, sleepy or "not themselves":

- Check to see if they're feeling ill, have abnormal vital signs, are in pain, or have a physical need (like hunger, cold or wet).

- Try the tips on the following page.

- If the person is still not themselves after 24 hours, consider contacting the health care provider.

Tips on Providing Relief at Home

A person with a sudden decrease in their activity should be watched carefully for signs of new illness, pain or a physical need. If these are not the cause, problem solve by thinking about the person's situation or routine.

If the person seems bored or is having trouble starting activities:

- Plan activities the person enjoys, and help them get started. Consider what they liked in the past, and adjust for what they can do now.

- Try music, singing, photo sorting, or folding clothes. If possible, take them for a walk, or play a game that encourages movement.

If the person seems tired or overwhelmed from too much activity:

- Keep the living area calm, quiet, and well lit.

- Keep activities short and allow time for rest.

- Avoid activities that are too hard or rushed, or places that are loud or unfamiliar.

- Keep a routine for sleep, meals and activities. If needed, try adjusting the schedule (for example, doing more physically demanding activities in the morning).

Other approaches:

- If the person has pain during certain activities, give a pain reliever like acetaminophen 2 hours before the activity.

- If the person is fearful of falling, make sure the home is safe and easy to move around in. See page 68 for more on falls and how to prevent them.

- Give the person plenty of time to do things and offer breaks when needed.

- If the person is not sleeping well, see pages 116–119 for more on daytime and nighttime sleep problems.

- If the person has signs of depression, including seeming sad or tearful most of the time, see page 58.

- If you think the decreased activity may be caused by a medication side effect, talk with a health care provider.

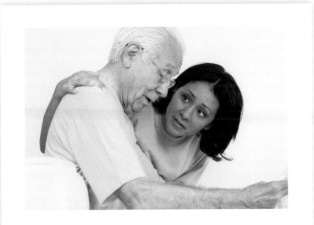

What to Watch Out For

- **Pressure ulcers or bed sores:** If the person sits or lies in the same position for too long, they can get skin wounds.

  - Encourage the person to move or shift weight often, or help them change positions.

  - Check the skin over bony areas for redness or sores.

  - See page 106 for more information.

- **Constipation:** If the person isn't moving around much, they're at risk for constipation.

  - See page 50 for more on how to prevent and treat constipation.

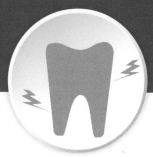

Dental Problems

Basic Facts

Good mouth care is often difficult for a person with middle or late stage dementia to handle themselves. They may forget how to use the toothbrush or forget to brush altogether, and they'll likely need your help to get the job done. This can be a challenge, especially if the person is scared, confused, or has mouth pain. But good mouth care is important, because cavities, tooth infections, mouth pain and even pneumonia can happen when teeth aren't cared for properly. Use the mouth care tips in this guide every day to keep teeth healthy and prevent problems.

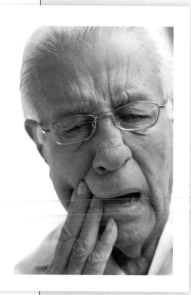

If the person has broken a tooth:

They should see a dentist right away. While you're waiting for an appointment, you can:

- Ask the person to rinse their mouth with warm water.
- If the tooth is bleeding, ask them to bite down on a clean piece of gauze or a wet tea bag.
- Place a cold compress on the cheek.
- Give acetaminophen (Tylenol) for pain.

While helping, never put your hands or fingers into the person's mouth.

Signs of a Possible Emergency

Consider taking the person to a dentist or health care provider office **SOON** if the person has any of these problems:

- **fever** with **swelling in the face or jaw**

Other Important Signs

Consider contacting a dentist by phone and/or setting up a medical visit **within 1–3 days if you notice any of the following:**

- **pain** with eating or when pressing on the tooth. Signs of mouth pain in persons with dementia who cannot explain how they feel include:

  - refusing to eat or drink
  - wincing in pain with chewing
  - avoiding foods that are hot or cold
  - biting their inner cheek or lip
  - drooling
  - acting differently during meals (angry, aggressive) or trying to bite you or other objects

- the mouth always seems dry and the tongue often covered with a white film
- **bad breath,** even with good mouth care
- **swelling, redness and/or a pimple on the gum** underneath a tooth
- a **tooth becomes darker** than the others
- **the person won't let you help with mouth care**

Tips on Providing Relief at Home

Here are general tips for a healthy mouth:

- Brush teeth twice a day with a fluoride toothpaste.
- If the person has red, inflamed gums, try brushing with an antibacterial rinse such as chlorhexidine (prescription needed) or Listerine Total Care Zero.
- Use a soft bristled toothbrush with a small head to get the hard-to-reach areas.
- Replace toothbrushes every 3–4 months.
- Clean between teeth daily with an interdental brush (This is easier than floss.)
- Have dental check-ups every 6–12 months.
- Drink water with fluoride.

If you're helping someone who is stressed by mouth care:

- Move and speak slowly; make eye contact.
- Make small talk about something they like.
- Explain what you'll be doing before you do it.
- Give the person something familiar to hold.
- Give encouragement and praise.
- Ask them if they want to try it themselves.
- Ask the person to tell you if anything you do hurts, and say that you'll stop if they have pain.
- Make mouth care a daily routine at the same times.
- If they still refuse, try again later.

If the person won't open their mouth:

- Stay calm and kind; explain what you're doing.
- Try gently touching their mouth, jaw or cheek with the toothbrush.
- If they're having trouble following directions, say "watch me" and show them how you open your mouth wide.
- Ask the person to smile, then brush the front teeth.
- Have the person sing a song they like and while opening wide, brush the back teeth.

What to Watch Out For

- **Mouth care at the end of life:** Brushing and flossing may not be possible.
  - Try wiping the teeth with an oral sponge soaked in a mouth rinse like Biotene or ACT
  - Offer fluids often
  - Apply lip ointment
- **Low fluid in the body (dehydration):** A person with mouth pain may not eat or drink well. Here are some signs of dehydration:
  - Dry mouth and tongue
  - Urinating very little
  - Fast heart beat
  - Slow, weak, or low energy

See page 98 for more on not eating or drinking.

If the person has dentures:

- Remove the dentures for at least 4–8 hours daily.
- Store them in a cup with water (to keep them from drying out).
- To clean the mouth: Wearing gloves, wrap gauze around your finger and dip in Listerine Total Care Zero or Biotene oral rinse. Massage gums, cheeks and roof of mouth. Then, have the person spit.
- To clean the dentures: Place dentures under running water and clean gently with a soft toothbrush. Never use toothpaste or fluoride on dentures.

Taking Care of Your Own Safety and Stress

- When helping with mouth care, wear gloves and never put your hands in their mouth. Use an interdental brush instead of regular floss.

See Chapter 3 for more ways to take care of yourself.

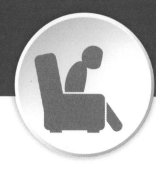

Depression

Basic Facts

Depression and dementia share many of the same symptoms, so it can be hard to identify depression in persons with dementia. When a person with dementia is depressed they may feel sad, hopeless, or tearful most of the time. They may also no longer enjoy doing the things they once did. Depression can be made worse by loss of a relative, having other medical conditions, pain or being alone. Other signs of depression include:

- Social isolation, not wanting to be around others
- Poor appetite
- Trouble sleeping
- Agitation (worried, restless)
- Irritability (angry, easily frustrated)
- Loss of energy
- Thoughts of death or suicide

Medications to treat depression often don't work well in persons with dementia. Medications also can have serious side effects. For these reasons, it's often best to try strategies to improve depression without medication first.

Signs of a Possible Emergency

Consider calling 911 or taking the person to an emergency department or health care provider office **SOON** if the person has any of these problems:

- **signs of dehydration** (see page 142 for more on dehydration)
- **you're worried the person may hurt themselves or others**
- **suicide warning signs: If the person talks about suicide,** especially if:
  - they have a plan for suicide,
  - they could carry out this plan,
  - they've decided when they're going to do it, and/or
  - they say they intend to do it

Other Important Signs

Consider contacting a health care provider by phone and/or setting up a medical visit **within 24 hours if you notice:**

- **severe depression symptoms** (like not eating or drinking, won't get out of bed or can't stop crying) even after you have tried the home care tips on the next page

If the person talks about suicide:

- Talk with them about it.
  See if they have any of the suicide warning signs.
- Decide if the person is in immediate danger. If so, call 911 and don't leave the person alone.
- Remove or lock up any dangerous items including guns, knives, and extra medicines.
- If the person isn't in immediate danger, talk to the health care provider soon for help.

Tips on Providing Relief at Home

If the person has signs of depression, try these strategies to help them feel better:

- Keep a routine for sleep, meals and activities. If needed, try adjusting the schedule (for example, doing more physically demanding activities in the morning).

- Keep the living area calm, quiet, and well lit.

- If possible, encourage time outdoors or sitting near a window every day.

- Encourage physical activity every day.

- If the person has early-stage dementia, encourage them to join an early-stage support group.

- Make a list of the person's favorite places, foods, music, people, and activities and offer at least one of these every day. Try talking about positive life events, hobbies or looking at old photos.

- Encourage activities where the person feels helpful and let them know they've helped.

- Offer reassurance that you love them and stay positive.

- Offer physical touch, like a hug or holding hands.

- Avoid activities, people, or places that are overwhelming. These may be activities that are too hard or rushed, or places that are loud, crowded or unfamiliar.

- Ask them about thoughts of death or suicide.

- If the person doesn't get better or gets worse, talk to a health care provider.

What to Watch Out For

- **Sudden outbursts of sadness or anger:** Dementia, especially frontotemporal type, can cause changes in the brain that lead to sudden emotional outbursts (crying, yelling) followed by times of normal mood. This is different from depression, which is sadness most of the time. If this is the case:
  - Pay attention to things that trigger the outbursts and problem solve.
  - Keep a calm daily routine.

- **Signs of suicide:** Aside from the suicide warning signs, you should be concerned if you notice any of the following, especially in a person with early-stage dementia:
  - Increased alcohol use
  - Stockpiling medications
  - Sudden interest in firearms
  - Elaborate good-byes
  - Rush to complete or revise a will

- **Other behavior challenges:** See the following pages for more tips on other problems that can come along with depression: agitation (page 30), anger (page 32), anxiety (page 34), not eating or drinking (page 98), and daytime and nighttime sleep problems (pages 116–119).

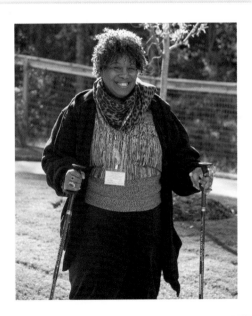

Tip: Encourage physical activity every day.

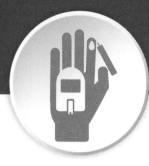

Diabetes Care

Basic Facts

Diabetes is a long-term illness in which blood sugar tends to be high due to too little insulin in the body. In type II diabetes (the most common kind) the body doesn't make enough insulin. Depending on the severity of the disease, blood sugar may be controlled by healthy diet, oral medication and/or insulin shots. In type I diabetes (which is less common and usually begins in childhood) the body doesn't make *any* insulin, so daily insulin shots are always needed. Both diabetes types require careful attention to diet, activity level, medications, stress and illness, as they can all impact blood sugar level. People with both dementia and diabetes may need daily help to take medicines, check and record blood sugar levels, and follow a healthy diet.

Diabetes that isn't well controlled can be dangerous. Blood sugar that stays high over years can lead to problems with the heart, kidneys, eyes, skin, circulation, and nerves. On the other hand, low blood sugar (a complication of treatment) can be an emergency, as it can lead to coma and even brain damage.

Signs of a Possible Emergency

Consider calling 911 or taking the person to an emergency department or health care provider office **SOON** if the person has any of these problems:

- passed out and can't be awakened
- blood sugar before eating in the morning is over 500 AND the person has any of these symptoms:
  - a fever (see page 70 for more on fever)
  - unusual confusion
  - unusual weakness

Other Important Signs

Consider contacting a health care provider by phone and/or setting up a medical visit **within 1–3 days if you notice:**

- very high and low blood sugars in the same day
- new or increased confusion with one or more blood sugar reading(s) less than 60 (even if they got better after a sugar boost)
- blood sugars over 350 for 2 or more days in a row
- new breaks in the skin on the feet (sores, cuts)
- new or increased redness, swelling, warmth, pain or discharge (fluid or pus) from any skin sore
- they won't take their diabetes medication
- the person isn't eating or is vomiting

If the person has low blood sugar and is awake:

- Give a sugar boost (like a glass of juice).
- After 15 minutes, recheck the blood sugar.
- If blood sugar is still below 60, give another sugar boost.
- Once the blood sugar is above 60, give a high protein snack (like yogurt or peanut butter) to keep the blood sugar from dropping again.
- Even if the person recovers quickly, consider calling their health care provider to report what happened.

If the person has low blood sugar and passes out:

- Call 911.
- Place a sugar boost (like maple syrup, jelly or glucose gel) inside the cheek.
- Check the blood sugar.

Tips on Providing Relief at Home

If the person forgets to take diabetes medications:

- In early dementia, try placing pills in a pill reminder box (with compartments for each day). That way you'll know what medicines were taken.

- For later stage dementia, caregivers should give the medications.

- Caregivers should give all insulin shots.

If the person refuses to take diabetes medications:

- If confused, try giving step-by-step instructions, like: "Put the pill in your mouth. That's good. Open your mouth and bring the cup to your lips like this..."

- If the person seems suspicious of the pill, don't argue. Take a break and try again in a few minutes.

- If you take medicine, take yours at the same time.

- Try playing a game. See how fast the person can take them.

- Talk to the health care provider about ways to decrease the number of medicines.

- For more on managing medications, see Chapter 7.

If the person gets sick:

- Help them rest and stay warm.

- If the person is not vomiting, continue diabetes medicines. If they are vomiting, contact a health care provider about what to do about their medicine.

- Check and record blood sugar several times a day along with any symptoms.

- Offer liquids frequently.

To prevent foot problems:

- Check the feet daily for sores or open skin, and apply moisturizer to feet daily after bathing.

- Always have the person wear socks and shoes (never barefoot).

- Be careful when cutting toenails. Avoid cutting them too short.

- See a health care provider for the care of any skin wounds. See page 114 for more on skin injury care and the signs of wound infection.

What to Watch Out For

Check and record blood sugar levels at home regularly (ask the health care provider how often) and look for:

- **Signs suggesting HIGH blood sugar:**
  - Flushed, red skin
  - Dry mouth
  - Fruity smelling breath
  - Frequent urination
  - Extreme thirst and hunger
  - Headache
  - Blurry vision
  - Nausea, vomiting
  - Seizures
- **Signs suggesting LOW blood sugar:**
  - Sweating
  - Shakiness, weakness
  - Increased anxiety or confusion
  - Lightheaded, dizzy feeling
  - Tingling around the mouth
  - Seizures
  - Slurred speech

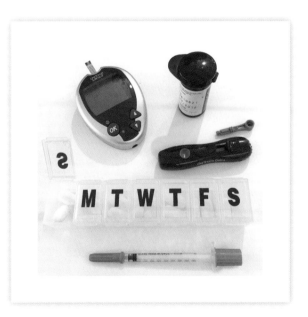

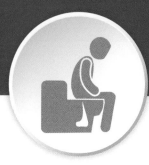

Diarrhea

Basic Facts

A single loose or runny stool is common after certain meals, depending on the individual. But, diarrhea—3 or more watery stools in a day—is most often caused by an infection with a virus or bacteria ("stomach bug"). Other causes include medications, abdominal surgery, problems with the intestines, stress and diet.

Diarrhea can cause significant problems for an older person with dementia, including skin problems, hygiene problems, and dehydration. This section will help you know what to watch for, how to treat at home, and when to get medical help.

Tip: Keep the belly light with foods like crackers, toast, and rice.

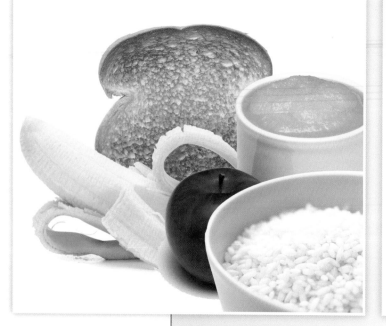

Signs of a Possible Emergency

Consider calling 911 or taking the person to an emergency department or health care provider office **SOON** if the person has any of these problems:

- severe belly pain, or belly pain that gets worse over time
- bloody, black, "tarry", or cranberry colored stool
- signs of dehydration
  (see page 142 for more on dehydration)
- signs of delirium
  (see page 48 for more on delirium)
- the person was in the hospital or on antibiotics in the past 2 months
- vital signs very different from usual, especially temperature above 100.5° F
  (see page 135 for how to measure vital signs)

Other Important Signs

Consider contacting a health care provider by phone and/or setting up a medical visit **within 1–3 days if you notice:**

- several days of no bowel movements, then watery stool
- diarrhea lasting more than 2 days
- more than 6 watery stools per day
- weight loss of 5 pounds within less than 2 weeks (even though the person is eating normally)
- greasy, grayish or very bad smelling stools
- low-grade fever for longer than 48 hours
  (see page 70 for more on fever)

Tips on Providing Relief at Home

Here are some things you can do at home for diarrhea:

- Offer plenty of fluids. Aim for the person to have between 4 and 6 cups of their favorite drinks each day (no alcohol or drinks high in caffeine).

  - Try sports drinks, like Gatorade. These drinks help put salt and sugar back in the body. Water and juices are also okay to drink.

  - Offer small sips every few minutes instead of big gulps all at once.

  - Try gelatins and popsicles.

  - Offer more than 6 cups of fluid daily if the diarrhea is severe or lasts more than 24 hours.

- Keep the belly light with foods like crackers, toast, and rice. Stay away from dairy products; they can sometimes worsen diarrhea.

- Try an over-the-counter medicine like loperamide (Imodium) to help stop the diarrhea, but keep in mind diarrhea helps rid the body of infection.

- If you've tried these tips and the person is still having diarrhea after 1 week, see a health care provider.

What to Watch Out For

- **Low fluid in the body (dehydration):** A person with dementia can quickly become dehydrated. Some signs of dehydration are:

  - Dry mouth and tongue

  - Urinating very little

  - Fast heart beat

  - Slow, weak, or low energy

  - If you've tried the tips on this page and the person still seems dehydrated, get medical help.

- **Skin rash or anal bleeding from wiping:** If this happens, try:

  - rinsing the anal area with warm water and patting dry instead of wiping with dry toilet paper

  - soaking the anal area in warm, shallow water (Sitz bath)

  - putting on a thin layer of a protective cream or ointment like A&D or Desitin

- **Sudden watery diarrhea after being constipated:** The person may have a hard ball of stool (called a "fecal impaction") with watery stool leaking around it.

  - Don't give medicine to stop the diarrhea.

  - Bring them to the health care provider who'll remove the hard stool.

Taking Care of Your Own Safety and Stress

When helping a person who has diarrhea:

- Wear gloves when helping with personal care.

- Clean toilet and sink areas well with germ-killing cleaners.

See Chapter 3 for more ways to take care of yourself.

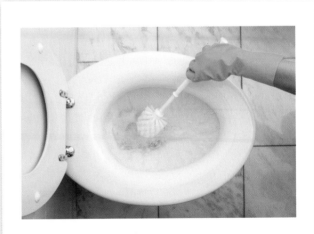

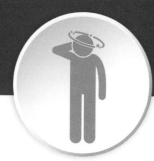

Dizziness

Basic Facts

"Dizzy" is a word that can mean many different things, including:

- A feeling of movement, as though you or the room were spinning, which is called vertigo. Vertigo commonly results from a problem with the brain, inner ear, or neck.

- Feeling as though you are about to pass out. This type of feeling often goes away when the person lies down. Common causes include heart problems, medications, and low blood pressure.

- Unsteadiness or loss of balance, often accompanied by fear of falling. Unsteadiness often results from a combination of problems and is common in people who are weak or frail.

- Fogginess, confusion, or another hard-to-describe feeling in your head that is uncomfortable but not painful. These are often as hard to diagnose as they are to describe.

Some dizziness can be a sign of a serious condition, such as a stroke, a problem with the heart, or low blood sugar for people with diabetes. More often, however, the cause is a combination of chronic problems and minor changes such as anxiety, depression, a virus, medication, dehydration, not eating enough, low blood pressure, drinking alcoholic beverages, lack of exercise or even wearing dirty eyeglasses.

Dizziness becomes more common as people get older, but persons with dementia may have a hard time describing it. As a caregiver, talk to a health care provider if you notice the person you care for suddenly seems uncomfortable or unstable when they stand, walk, or turn their head, as this may be a clue that they're dizzy. Also, pay careful attention to safety if the person seems at risk of falling.

If the person develops severe dizziness and vomiting:

- Have them sit down and reassure them that you are there.

- Give them something to throw up into, then help them rinse their mouth out with water.

- Encourage the person to lie still.

- Check vital signs and look for signs of weakness on one side or slurred speech that might suggest a stroke (see page 120).

- If anything makes you uncomfortable, call a health care provider or 911.

Signs of a Possible Emergency

Consider calling 911 or taking the person to an emergency department or health care provider office **SOON** if the person has any of these problems:

- New or worsening **chest pain or trouble breathing,** especially if accompanied by feeling the person is about to pass out (or passes out).

- A heartbeat or pulse that is **unusually rapid, irregular, or very slow.**

- **Loss of vision, double vision, or weakness in the face, arm, or leg.**

- The person is so lightheaded on standing that they **fall, pass out, or feel they might fall or pass out.**

- The person has **diabetes, gets weak or woozy, and then passes out.**

Other Important Signs

Consider contacting a health care provider by phone and/or setting up a medical visit **within 1–3 days if you notice:**

- Gradually increasing dizziness along with worsening hearing loss in one ear

- New lightheadedness on standing

- Spinning sensation when the person rolls over in bed, bends over and straightens up, or turns their head

- Dizziness after starting a new medication

- New dizziness accompanied by balance difficulty

- New dizziness along with fever

- The person has diabetes and frequently complains of dizziness

Tips on Providing Relief at Home

In certain cases, dizziness has a specific cause that can be treated, such as a medicine side effect, dehydration, a heart problem, or anxiety. However, more often dizziness in older persons doesn't have a single cause or cure. Below are general tips to decrease symptoms and manage dizziness at home:

- Encourage plenty of fluids and a healthy diet.

- Encourage physical activity. This can improve dizziness that is due to weakness or low blood pressure.

- For certain types of vertigo, especially those caused by head movement, specific exercises can help. Consult the health care provider or physical therapist for the best regimen.

- Encourage healthy sleep habits, as lack of sleep can make dizziness worse.

- Dizziness symptoms can often be improved by improving vision. Encourage the person to wear clean glasses, get regular eye exams, and consider cataract surgery if relevant.

- Dizziness medications usually create more side effects than relief in older persons, especially those with dementia; so, non-medication treatments are usually best. Ginger tea is safe and will improve some kinds of dizziness.

If the person feels like they might pass out:

- Help them to lie down and raise their legs about 12 inches above their heart level. Use a recliner or prop their legs up with pillows on a couch or bed.

- If they can't lie down, try to help them to a chair and have them put their head between their legs.

- Loosen any tight clothing.

- If the person has diabetes and you think they might have low blood sugar, get them a food or drink with sugar in it (like juice) and check their blood sugar. See page 60 for more on diabetes.

- Check the pulse and blood pressure.

- If the person has abnormal vital signs, doesn't feel back to normal within a few minutes, or has any other symptoms (see Signs of a Possible Emergency) consider getting medical care right away.

- For more information, see page 104 on passing out.

What to Watch Out For

- **Falls:** Dizziness can make the person more prone to falls. If the person is dizzy when standing, have them get up slowly and use a walker or sturdy piece of furniture to steady themselves. See page 68 for more on falls and fall prevention.

- **Weakness:** Sometimes the person who is dizzy will stop moving for fear of making the dizziness worse or falling. Over time, they can lose strength and stamina. Consult a physical therapist for ways to stay active and safe.

- **Dehydration:** Dizziness may cause the person to not drink enough fluids. In addition to encouraging small amounts of fluids frequently, the person may need a medication for nausea and/or intravenous fluids. See page 142 for more on dehydration.

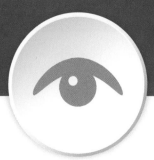

Eye Problems

Basic Facts

Eye problems can range from bothersome to emergencies. Here are common causes of eye problems:

- **Infections ("pink eye") or allergies:** Red, itchy, swollen eyes with thick discharge can be caused by a virus (especially if the person has a cold), bacterial infection, or allergy.

- **Droopy eyelids:** With age, the eyelids can droop and cause the eye to become red and dry.

- **Bleeding in the white of the eyeball:** Broken blood vessels in the white of the eyeball can happen from rubbing the eye, coughing, sneezing or vomiting. Although it looks scary, it's painless, causes no problems with vision, and gets better on its own.

- **Stys and eyelid swelling:** Stys (small, painful, pimple-like bumps on the eyelid) and eyelid swelling can usually be treated at home.

- **More urgent eye problems:** These include eye injuries or scratches to the eyes' surface, eye pressure problems, or problems with the nerves or blood flow to the eye. These problems will often cause pain and/or changes to the person's vision and should be treated right away.

Tip: To prevent infection, wash your hands before helping the person.

Signs of a Possible Emergency

Consider calling 911 or taking the person to an emergency department or health care provider office **SOON** if the person has any of these problems:

- **sudden vision loss or change in vision** (blurry vision, double vision, light flashes, "floaters")

- **any severe eye pain,** especially with headache, changes in vision, nausea or vomiting

- **light bothers the eye(s)**

- **change in size of the pupil** (black part of eye)

- the person **feels like there is something in the eye but can't open the eye**

Other Important Signs

Consider contacting a health care provider by phone and/or setting up a medical visit **within 1–3 days if you notice:**

- any **cut, scratch, injury to, or chemicals in the eye**

- **red or pink eye with an oozy or sticky drainage or crusting**

- **a red ring around the colored part of the eye** (see an ophthalmologist)

- **eyelid swelling** that doesn't go away after home treatment

Tips on Providing Relief at Home

To prevent infection, wash your hands before helping the person with eye care.

If the person needs eye drops to treat an eye problem:

- Don't touch the tip of the eye drop container to the eye.
- If the person is fearful of eye drops:
  - Help the person to lie comfortably on a bed or couch with their eyes closed.
  - Place the drops into the corner of the closed eye, near the nose.
  - The drops will seep into the eyes and then go in fully once the eyes open.
  - If the person doesn't like cold drops, ask the health care provider if the drops can be warmed by placing the bottle under warm running water for 10–15 seconds.
  - If you have trouble getting the drops into the eye due to shaky or weak hands, ask a pharmacist about products that can help.
  - If the person is very upset about the drops, don't force it. Try again later.
  - If the person is missing many doses of drops, talk to the health care provider.

If the person has a sty or eyelid swelling:

- Make a warm compress by wetting a folded washcloth with warm water, wringing out any extra water, and placing it on and off the affected eyelid throughout the day.
- Gently scrub the eyelid with a small amount of baby shampoo mixed with warm water. Use a clean washcloth to massage the lid while the eye is closed.
- If the swelling gets worse or doesn't get better after 3 days, bring the person to their health care provider.

If the person has something (like an eyelash or dirt) in the eye:

- Encourage the person not to rub or push on the eye.
- Encourage the person to blink.
- Try rinsing the eye with water a few times.
- If you feel able, wash your hands and lift the upper and lower eyelids to look for the object. Don't touch the eyeball with anything (cotton swab, tweezers).
- If still painful or stuck, get medical help.
- If a chemical (like a household cleaner) went in the eye, flush it out with cool running water for 15–30 minutes, then get medical help.

If the person has bleeding into the white part of the eye and can see fine:

- Usually the problem clears up on its own in a week or two.
- A cold compress may speed healing.
- See a health care provider if the bleeding happened after an injury, if the person is on a blood thinner, or if the person develops any of the warning signs of a possible emergency.

See page 126 for more on vision problems.

Taking Care of Your Own Safety and Stress

If the person has an eye infection:

- Wash your hands well with soap and water before and after helping with eye care. Try not to touch your own face or eyes.
- Avoid sharing towels, pillows or other personal items.

See Chapter 3 for more ways to take care of yourself.

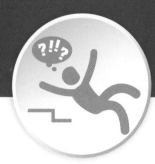

Falls and Falling

Basic Facts

Falls are very common in older persons, especially those with dementia, and can be a major source of worry for caregivers. Falls often happen for a combination of reasons, including:

- **Changes to the body.** Poor vision, balance, reflexes and strength are common in older persons. When combined with feeling worried, confused or problems knowing what is safe, falls can happen easily.

- **A new or worsening illness.** A fall can be the first sign of a new problem like infection or stroke.

- **Medication reactions.** Medications can cause side effects like sleepiness and changes in blood pressure that make a person less steady. Talk to a health care provider about new medicines or medicines that were not taken properly as possible causes of a fall.

- **Safety hazards.** Poor lighting, lack of hand rails, throw rugs and unsafe shoes can increase the risk of falls.

Signs of a Possible Emergency

Consider calling 911 or taking the person to an emergency department or health care provider office **SOON** if the person has any of these problems:

- passing out
- new confusion or trouble staying awake
- seizure either before, during, or after a fall
- a cut that needs stitches or bleeding that you can't stop
- a change in the ability to move, stand or walk
- a possible broken bone
- severe headache
- new shortness of breath
- vomiting more than once in the 24 hours after a fall
- new neck, abdominal or chest pain
- vital signs very different from usual (see page 135 for how to measure vital signs)

Other Important Signs

Consider contacting a health care provider by phone and/or setting up a medical visit **within 1–3 days if you notice:**

- **falling more than once or more than usual,** even if the person seems fine after each fall
- the person seemed fine for a while after a fall but now just **doesn't seem their normal self**
- the person seems **more unsteady than usual,** even if they're not falling, and you're worried about keeping them safe

If the person just fell:

- Try to stay calm.
- If the person is passed out or you think they may have a serious injury, **call 911.**
- Don't move them or help them up until you know it's safe.
- If possible, ask "Do you hurt anywhere?" Ask about each body part.
- If they can't answer, watch the way they move for signs of pain.
- Touch them to check for injury. Check the head, neck, shoulders, wrists, hips, and knees.
- If they seem okay, help them up slowly or call for help.

Tips on Providing Relief at Home

If the person falls but seems okay (especially if they got up on their own):

- Encourage them to rest comfortably in a chair or bed.
- If they're upset, reassure them. Calming music, their favorite show, or another distraction can help.
- Take care of any minor cuts or injuries (see page 114).
- Keep an eye out for new problems. See the "What to Watch Out For" box (right).

To help prevent future falls:

- Talk to the health care provider about possible medication side effects, including over-the-counter medicines.
- Have the person's vision checked.
- Ask the health care provider to check for blood pressure changes when the person goes from sitting to standing, since this can cause faintness and falls.
- Think about an exercise program to gain strength and balance.
- Do a home safety check to make the home as safe and comfortable as possible.

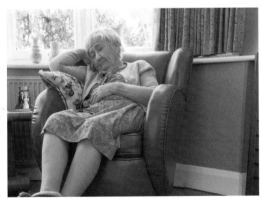

Tip: Do a home safety check to make the home as safe and comfortable as possible.

What to Watch Out For

- **New illness:** In the hours and days after a fall, keep watch for any new signs or symptoms like fever, cough, rash or diarrhea.

- **Injuries:** Serious injuries like broken bones or bleeding inside the body may not be obvious right way. Over the next 24–48 hours, get medical attention for:
  - new confusion or trouble staying awake
  - new weakness
  - new trouble walking or standing
  - new chest, abdominal or severe head pain
  - shortness of breath
  - vomiting more than once in 24 hours after a fall

- **More falls:** If the person is more unsteady than usual, they're likely to fall again. Stay close by and encourage rest until they're back to normal.

Taking Care of Your Own Safety and Stress

To prevent getting hurt when lifting the person off the floor:

- Call for help if you need it.
- If the person can do it, ask them to hold onto a sturdy object like a large chair and pull themselves up while you steady them.
- If you must lift, use your legs and not your back, keeping the person close to you.

See Chapter 3 for more ways to take care of yourself.

Fever

Basic Facts

Fever is increased body temperature. Although a fever by itself is usually not dangerous, it can be a sign of serious illness. The most common causes of high fever in older adults are respiratory infections (such as the flu or pneumonia), urinary tract infections, and skin infections. Low grade fevers can be caused by other things, such as being in a hot room, being constipated, or agitation.

Older persons tend to have lower "usual" body temperatures than children and younger adults; so, for the average older person, a temperature over 99.0° F is often considered a fever. If you know the person's normal body temperature, an increase of between 1.2° F and 2.0° F is probably a fever. Because temperature changes so small can be hard to detect by touching the skin, it's good to have a reliable thermometer and use it whenever you think the person may be sick.

In general, the higher the temperature, the more concerned you should be about a serious illness. In older persons, temperatures under 100.5° F are usually considered "low grade," and temperatures over 101° F may represent an emergency. In any case, fever should be watched carefully and reported to the person's health care provider.

Signs of a Possible Emergency

Consider calling 911 or taking the person to an emergency department or health care provider office **SOON** if the person has any of these problems:

- One temperature reading of **higher than 101° F**, especially with any of the following:
  - **trouble breathing**
  - **unusual weakness, sleepiness, or confusion**
  - **nausea, vomiting, or diarrhea**
  - **skin infection signs** including redness, warmth, and tenderness (see page 115)
  - **urine infection signs** including pain with urination or lower belly pain (see page 124)
  - one or more **swollen, red, tender joints** (like the knee, elbow, shoulder, or hip)
  - the person has a **chronic illness** (like HIV or chronic lung disease) or is on a **medicine that weakens the immune system** (like prednisone or cancer chemotherapy)

Other Important Signs

Consider contacting a health care provider by phone and/or setting up a medical visit **within 1–3 days if the person has a fever under 101° F AND:**

- **you're concerned** about the person's illness
- the **fever has lasted for over 24 hours**, even if the person seems okay
- **the person has abnormal vital signs** (see page 135 for how to measure vital signs)
- the person has a **chronic illness** (like HIV or chronic lung disease) or is on a **medicine that weakens the immune system** (like prednisone or cancer chemotherapy)

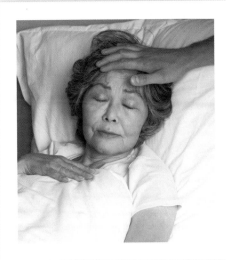

Tip: Measure and record the person's temperature every few hours.

Tips on Providing Relief at Home

To help the person feel more comfortable when they have a fever:

- Measure and record the person's temperature every few hours. See page 139 for more on how to measure temperature.

- Give a fever-reducing medicine like acetaminophen (Tylenol) or ibuprofen (Motrin or Advil). Talk to the person's provider about which is best.

- If the person has chills or feels cold, offer a light sheet or jacket.

- If the person feels hot, take off any extra layers of clothing, turn on a fan, put a cold washcloth on the skin, or offer a cool bath.

- Offer more fluid than usual (8 or more cups each day). Keep drinks they enjoy within reach and encourage frequent sips.

To prevent respiratory (cold and flu-type) and stomach illnesses:

- See the health care provider for regular care and for flu and pneumonia shots.

- Wash hands often.

- Avoid other people who are sick.

- Encourage healthy eating, sleep and physical activity.

What to Watch Out For

- **Low fluid in the body (dehydration):** A person with fever can quickly become dehydrated. Some signs of dehydration are:

  - Dry mouth and tongue
  - Urinating very little
  - Fast heart beat
  - Slow, weak, or low energy

  See page 99 for tips on how to encourage fluid intake. If you've tried these tips, but the person still seems dehydrated or is getting worse, get medical help.

- **Falls:** When a person with dementia has a fever, they're often unsteady, making falls more likely. If they're unsteady:

  - Encourage the person to not get out of bed or up from a chair without help.
  - If they are up and moving, stay close by or give them something to hold on to.
  - See page 68 for more on falls.

Taking Care of Your Own Safety and Stress

- If the person has an illness that may be contagious, wash your hands often. If the person is coughing, have the person wear a mask. If they can't wear one, wear one yourself.

- If you're helping with wound care, vomit or bathroom accidents, use disposable gloves.

- Get your flu shot each year.

- A good diet, regular exercise, and plenty of sleep will help you stay healthy.

See Chapter 3 for more ways to take care of yourself.

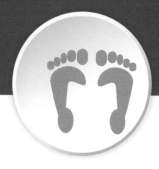

Foot Problems

Basic Facts

Persons with memory problems need help to keep their feet healthy for numerous reasons. Poor balance and dexterity make foot injuries more likely, and people with diabetes or circulation problems require particularly careful care. Additionally, the person may not be able to communicate about foot pain. For these reasons, it's important to have a daily foot care routine that includes proper grooming and checking for any problems.

Foot pain. Foot pain is common in older persons and may be even more common in persons with dementia, although the person may not be able to say what is bothering them. Common causes of foot pain include arthritis and uncomfortable shoes.

Changes to the shape of the foot or toes. These are common and can lead to pain and to difficulty finding comfortable footwear. Foot changes include:

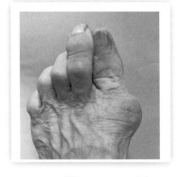

**Hammer Toe
and Bunion**

- Hammer toes—toes that are bent downward.
- Bunion—a change in the angle of the front of the foot, in which the big toe is at an angle creating a bump on the inside of the base of the big toe.
- Callouses and/or corns—hard bumps of thickened skin, often due to rubbing.

Treatment may include changing footwear, padding problem areas, shoe inserts, foot exercises, pain medicine, and/or surgery.

Toenail fungus. This chronic but usually non-serious infection causes nails to be thickened and discolored.

Ingrown toenail. This is an inflammation along the side of a toenail, usually involving the big toe. Ingrown nails are often caused by clipping the edge of the toenail too short, so that a corner of nail grows into the skin, causing pain and redness. Ingrown toenails can often be treated at home (see next page).

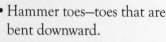

Signs of a Possible Emergency

Consider calling 911 or taking the person to an emergency department or health care provider office **SOON** if the person has any of these problems:

- A toe with an ulcer has become black, swollen, or draining pus.
- An object (such as a nail or a piece of glass) is lodged in the bottom of the foot.
- A wound is bleeding a lot.
- A wound shows signs of infection (redness, swelling, pus) and the person has a fever.

Other Important Signs

Consider contacting a health care provider by phone and/or setting up a medical visit **within 1-3 days if you notice:**

- New changes to the shape of toes or feet
- New foot pain
- New swelling, redness or a burning sensation on the feet
- Any new break in the skin of the foot, especially if the person has diabetes or poor circulation (see page 92 for more on foot wounds)

Tips on Providing Relief at Home

If the person has foot pain, foot deformities, and/or raw areas where skin is rubbed:

- Replace any shoes that are rubbing skin or causing pain; get better fitting shoes.

- Ask your pharmacy about non-prescription pads to cushion sore spots.

- If the person has pain, consider giving an oral pain medicine, like acetaminophen (Tylenol), before providing foot care.

If the person has an ingrown toenail:

- Soak area in warm water for 15 minutes 3–4 times a day to reduce swelling and tenderness.

- If the person has pain, consider giving an oral pain medicine like acetaminophen (Tylenol).

- Keep the area free from being rubbed by tight footwear.

- If the area doesn't improve, worsens, or if you notice pus, seek medical attention.

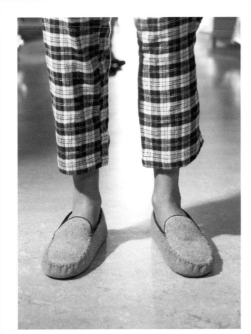

Tip: Encourage wearing socks and shoes or slippers.

To prevent foot problems:

- Check the feet every day for blisters, cuts, sores, bruises, redness, or swelling. Any change should be treated at home and if necessary, reported to a health care provider.

- Wash feet regularly. Use warm water, mild soap, and a washcloth. Encourage the person to wash him or herself if possible. If the person requires help, take care to avoid causing pain. Be sure to wash between the toes. Rinse thoroughly and pat dry with a towel, including between the toes. Then apply lotion to the tops and bottoms of each foot, avoiding lotion between the toes.

- Trim toenails regularly. If the person has diabetes or circulation problems, consider having their toenails trimmed by a health care professional.

- Encourage the person to always wear socks and shoes or slippers. Going barefoot even in the house increases the risk of injury.

- Choose sturdy, comfortable shoes of a breathable material with a non-slip sole.

  - Make sure the toes are not crowded in the front of the shoe (called the "toe box"). Avoid pointy shoes.

  - Always wear socks with shoes. Smooth out any sock wrinkles when putting shoes over socks.

  - Make sure the shoes are not too tight; check for signs that skin is being rubbed.

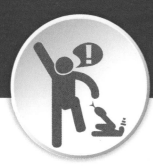

Hallucinations and Delusions

Basic Facts

Hallucinations happen when a person sees, hears, smells, tastes or feels something that isn't really there. For example, the person may feel insects crawling on the skin or see a face in the curtains. Often in persons with dementia the "hallucination" is poor vision or hearing, causing the person to mistake something real (like a mirror reflection) for something imagined (like a stranger in the house). On the other hand, true hallucinations are common in Lewy body dementia and can also occur during delirium.

Delusions happen when a person believes something that isn't true, such as believing a caregiver is stealing from them. Delusions are more common than hallucinations for persons with Alzheimer's type dementia. Both can be distressing and dangerous.

Sometimes, hallucinations and delusions are caused by dementia. However, they can also be caused by a new medical problem (like infection or stroke), medications or alcohol. For these reasons, new or worsening hallucinations or delusions, especially when they come along with other medical symptoms, should always be brought to a health care provider's attention.

Signs of a Possible Emergency

Consider calling 911 or taking the person to an emergency department or health care provider office **SOON** if the person has any of these problems:

- **signs of delirium** (see page 48 for more on delirium)

- **hallucinations involving more than one sense** (like imagined sounds and smells in addition to visions)

- **sudden vision loss in one or both eyes**

- **the person may hurt themselves or others**

- **vital signs very different from usual**, especially temperature over 101° F (see page 135 for how to measure vital signs)

Other Important Signs

Consider contacting a health care provider by phone and/or setting up a medical visit **within 1–3 days if you notice:**

- **new or worsening hallucinations or delusions** (lasting longer, harder to console)

- **difficulty keeping the person or others safe**

- **difficulty keeping the person calm or distracted**

If the person is upset by a hallucination or delusion:

- Try to stay calm and reassuring.

- Distract the person from the upsetting thought.

- If possible, remove any objects or sounds that are upsetting them.

- If the person is violent and you're unable to calm them, step away and get help.

- See the next page for more details and ideas on what to say and do.

Tips on Providing Relief at Home

Some people with hallucinations or delusions (especially people with Lewy body dementia) are not bothered by them. Many are, however. If the person you care for suffers from upsetting hallucinations and/or delusions, here are some tips to try:

Offer calm reassurance.

- Don't argue with the person about what they see, hear, or believe.

- Reassure the person with kind words. You might say: "I'm here. I'll protect you."

- Reassure the person with a gentle touch, but ask first. You might say: "Would it help if I held your hand?"

Use distraction.

- Try bringing them to a well-lit room and offer an activity they enjoy (like music).

- If they won't leave the room, you might say: "I know you're worried. Would you like me to walk with you for a while?"

- If they're worried about having lost something, you might say: "Before we look, why don't we take a break and have some ice cream?"

If the person asks you about what they're experiencing:

- Try being honest. You might say: "I know that you see something, but I don't see it."

- Try "fixing" the imagined problem. For example, if they see snakes, pretend to kill them; if they believe there are people in the house, say they went home to bed.

- Show you understand their feelings. You might say: "I know this is scary for you."

If the person can't be distracted, see if there's something around them causing distress.

- If the person sees a face in the curtains, try taking the curtains down.

- If the person sees holes where there are dark floor tiles, try putting a rug over them.

- If the person hears noises, check for sounds coming from a TV, radio, furnace, or air conditioning unit.

- If the person misplaces an item and believes someone is stealing from them, have extras on hand to replace the missing item.

If the person is violent (hitting, pushing):

- Keep dangerous items (knives, guns, heavy objects) locked or out of the home.

- Back away to give them space. Call for help if you need it.

- See page 32 for more on anger and tips to prevent it.

If the person is agitated, irritable, restless, or seems uncomfortable:

- Look for signs of pain, hunger, needing to use the bathroom or sleepiness.

- See page 30 for more on agitation and how to prevent it.

Taking Care of Your Own Safety and Stress

Taking care of someone with hallucinations or delusions can be stressful. Try not to take their behavior personally and have a plan to keep yourself safe.

See Chapter 3 for more ways to take care of yourself.

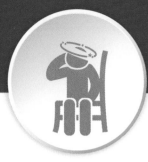

Head Injury

Basic Facts

When an older person falls or hits their head, they may get a bump, bruise or cut on the face or scalp that needs care. What medical providers worry most about, however, is invisible bleeding or bruising inside the brain, which is not very common but can be life-threatening. For this reason, most providers recommend older persons with even a minor head injury be brought to the emergency room to get a head scan (CT scan) and to be watched closely.

For many with dementia, however, a trip to the ER can be so challenging it may cause more harm than good. In this case, keeping careful watch on the person after a minor head injury and knowing what emergency signs to look for may be a better choice.

If the person passes out:

Try to stay calm. Most people wake up soon.
Call 911 and while waiting for help:

- Check for breathing and pulse.
- If there's no breathing or no pulse, and resuscitation is part of the care plan, start CPR (cardiopulmonary resuscitation). To learn CPR, call the American Heart Association at 1-877-242-4277 or visit www.cpr.heart.org.
- If they're breathing and have a pulse:
  - lie them on their side to prevent choking (don't move them if they may have a neck injury)
  - loosen tight clothes
  - put pressure on any bleeding
  - cover them with a blanket if it's cold
  - after they "come to," see page 114 for tips on how to check for injuries

If the person fell:

Don't move them until you know it's safe.
See page 68 for more on falls.

Signs of a Possible Emergency

Consider calling 911 or taking the person to an emergency department or health care provider office **SOON** if the person has any of these problems:

- passing out
- a fall from high up (more than 5 stairs or 3 feet)
- blood inside ear(s), bruising behind ear(s) or under eyes
- a cut that needs stitches, or that won't stop bleeding
- new or worsened confusion more than 20–30 minutes after the injury
- new or worsened weakness, trouble speaking or walking
- new problems with vision, or severe headache
- vomiting more than once in 24 hours after injury
- new sleepiness or trouble waking the person up
- vital signs very different from usual, especially slow breathing rate or high blood pressure (see page 135 for how to measure vital signs)

Other Important Signs

Consider contacting a health care provider by phone and/or setting up a medical visit **within 1–3 days if the person hit their head AND:**

- is on a **blood thinner** such as warfarin (Coumadin), rivaroxaban (Xarelto), epixaban (Eliquis), dabigatran (Pradaxa), or enoxaparin (Lovenox)
- has a headache that lasts more than 24 hours
- feels nauseated for more than 24 hours, even if they don't vomit
- has new or worsening irritability or bad temper
- is not eating or eating less than usual
- has new or worsening problems sleeping

Tips on Providing Relief at Home

For the first 24 hours after a head injury, it's important to keep a close eye on the person. During this time, you should:

- Stay home with them. Don't let them drive a car or bathe alone.

- Avoid things like alcohol and narcotic pain medicines that can make the person sleepy or confused.

- Check on them every two hours while they're awake, watching especially for any of the signs listed on the previous page.

- It can be normal for the person to have an upset stomach, or even vomit once after a head injury. If so, keep the belly light. Offer clear liquids, like jello, juice, or Gatorade. If they do well with these, move to soup broth, and then try a light sandwich.

If the person has a cut that is bleeding:

- Apply pressure with clean gauze or dressing.

- If the bleeding does not stop in 15–20 minutes, consider seeing a health care provider for stitches.

If the person has a bump, knot or bruise on their head, or a black eye:

- Apply ice (wrapped in a towel) on and off every 20–30 minutes for the first 24 hours. A bag of frozen peas or other vegetables works well if you don't have an ice pack.

- Don't put heat on the head in the first 24 hours as it may make swelling worse.

If the person seems physically okay, but is shaken up or upset:

- Be reassuring. Help them sit in a comfortable chair with their feet up.

- Try playing soothing music, or put on a favorite television show or movie.

If the person has a headache or other pain:

- For temporary pain relief, use acetaminophen (Tylenol) or another pain medication recommended by their provider.

- If possible, don't give narcotic pain medications like oxycodone or morphine. These stronger pain medicines can make a person sleepy or confused, making it hard to tell if there's a complication from the injury.

- Don't give aspirin, BC, or Goody powders as these medications can make bleeding worse.

Taking Care of Your Own Safety and Stress

To prevent getting hurt when lifting the person off the floor:

- Call for help if you need it.

- If possible, have them pull up using a sturdy object, like a chair, while you're there for support.

- If you must lift them, use your legs and not your back, keeping the person close to you.

See Chapter 3 for more ways to take care of yourself.

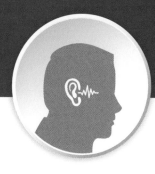

Hearing Problems

Basic Facts

For the person with dementia, hearing trouble can have a big impact, as it can make confusion worse and lead to worry and sadness. It can also make the person less able to do things they once enjoyed. For this reason, it's important to do what you can to treat and manage a hearing problem.

Most hearing problems develop slowly, over years. If a hearing problem develops quickly, the problem could be an ear infection, injury to the eardrum (from loud noise or poking with a Q-tip, for example) a buildup of earwax, or a sudden problem with blood supply to the inner ear or brain. If the person suddenly can't hear, especially if they're also having other sudden problems like weakness or numbness, they should get medical attention right away, as this can be a sign of stroke.

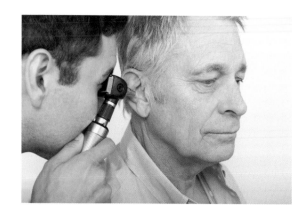

Signs of a Possible Emergency

Consider calling 911 or taking the person to an emergency department or health care provider office **SOON** if the person has any of these problems:

- **sudden hearing loss** in one or both ears

- **blood** coming from the person's ear

- **pain** in or around one of the ears and a **temperature over 101° F**

- **injury** from an object placed in the ear

- **something stuck in the ear** (like a bead or an insect)

- **vital signs very different from usual** (see page 135 for how to measure vital signs)

Other Important Signs

Consider contacting a health care provider by phone and/or setting up a medical visit **within 1–3 days if you notice:**

- **pain or stuffiness in or around the ear** that lasts for more than a day

- **discharge** (like fluid or pus) is coming from the ear

Tips on Providing Relief at Home

Sometimes hearing loss that happens slowly goes unnoticed or is mistaken for worsening dementia. Here are some signs that the person should have their hearing tested:

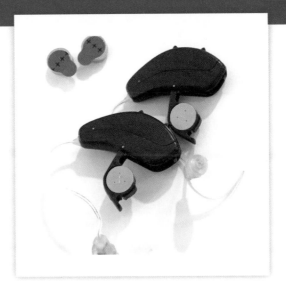

- trouble hearing when there's background noise, when several people are talking at once, or when the sound is high-pitched (such as a woman or child's voice)

- asking for questions to be repeated or for the TV to be turned up

- speaking out of turn or answering questions in ways that don't make sense

- complaining of ringing or hissing noises

If you're having trouble communicating with a person with hearing problems:

- Keep the room well lit, and speak so the person can see your mouth; this allows the person to lip read and/or get clues from your facial expressions.

- If one ear is better than the other, stand slightly to the side of the good ear.

- Speak clearly and slowly with a low-pitched voice.

- Keep sentences short and pause between statements to give the person time to understand.

- When starting a conversation, address the person by name, so they know you're talking to them.

- When possible, avoid background noises (like TV or side conversations).

- Avoid sudden changes in topic or interrupting others.

- Don't shout. This changes the voice and can make lip reading more difficult.

- If a hearing aid is not an option or if the person won't wear it, try an assisted listening device sold at many electronics stores. This can help with conversations, TV watching, and more.

If the person has a hearing aid:

- Work with a hearing specialist to ensure the hearing aid is adjusted for the person's needs.

- Even with a hearing aid, the person may still have trouble hearing. Use the tips on this page to help with communication.

- To save battery life, take hearing aids out before bedtime and turn them off when not in use. Always have replacement batteries on hand.

- Turn the hearing aid off or down in times when background noise is loud.

If the person has hearing loss due to earwax:

- Unless instructed by a health care provider, avoid putting anything inside the ear canal. See a provider for help with earwax removal.

If the person has ear pain and is being treated by a health care provider:

- Use acetaminophen (Tylenol) or another pain reliever recommended by the provider.

- Apply a warm washcloth or heating pad to the outside of the ear.

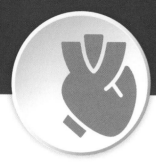

Heart Failure

Basic Facts

Heart failure, often referred to as congestive heart failure, is a common condition. When the heart doesn't work as well as it's supposed to, it has trouble pumping the blood as well as it used to. Causes include high blood pressure, diabetes, heart disease, certain medications or heavy alcohol use.

When the heart doesn't pump well, fluid backs up in other parts of the body. The person may experience difficulty with breathing because fluid may be in their lungs or because the body may not be getting enough blood from the heart. Swelling can appear in the legs, ankles, feet, and/or the abdomen. Fatigue is common as well.

Treatment for heart failure focuses on keeping the person in good health by having them exercise, lose weight, take their prescribed medications, eat a low salt diet, and quit smoking and/or drinking alcohol. Medications are used to help the heart pump better, keep blood pressure low, and remove excess fluid from the body.

Closely monitoring the person's weight for changes is an important part of treatment. Health care providers consider it a warning sign if weight goes up three or more pounds in a day or 5 or more pounds in a week.

Signs of a Possible Emergency

Consider calling 911 or taking the person to an emergency department or health care provider office **SOON** if the person with heart failure has any of these problems:

- New shortness of breath while sitting
- Chest pain and...
  - The person passes out (even if only for a few seconds)
  - Effort or exercise makes the pain worse
  - The person is sweating, nauseated, or vomiting
  - Vital signs are abnormal, especially if breathing rate is increased, pulse is markedly different from normal (either faster or slower), or blood pressure is abnormally low
- Heart beat is over 120 beats per minute or under 45 beats per minute, especially if the person feels weak or dizzy or has chest pain

Other Important Signs

Consider contacting a health care provider by phone and/or setting up a medical visit **within 1–3 days if you notice:**

- New coughing and/or wheezing
- Rapid increase in leg or belly swelling
- Feeling lightheaded, dizzy, or passing out
- New or worsening confusion
- New shortness of breath while active
- Weight gain of 2–3 pounds (or more) within 24 hours or 5 pounds (or more) within 5 days
- Shortness of breath at night (relieved by sitting or propping up)

Tips on Providing Relief at Home

There are many things you can do to manage heart failure at home:

- Monitor the person's vital signs, especially their blood pressure and pulse.

- Weigh the person daily and write it down. Report weight gain to the health care provider.

- Help the person maintain a healthy lifestyle by exercising, avoiding smoking and alcohol use, reducing salt intake, and getting rest.

- Remind the person to take their medications as prescribed.

If the person has breathing difficulties:

- Help them get into a better body position:

  - If seated, help them lean forward and rest their elbows on their knees or a table.

  - If standing and there is no place to sit down, help them rest against a wall and lean forward with their hands on their thighs.

  - If unable to get out of bed, help them sit as upright as possible.

- If the person tolerates it, try blowing cool air over their face with a fan.

- Try distracting them with calming music.

- See page 40 for more on breathing problems, including deep breathing techniques.

If the person becomes short of breath when doing everyday activities:

- Take breaks often. For example, encourage rest after putting on each piece of clothing.

- Use assistive devices, such as a walker or a shower chair.

- Encourage them to use the bathroom regularly to avoid having to rush to get to the bathroom.

- Place chairs throughout the home to provide a rest stop while walking.

Preventing Infections

People with heart failure are more susceptible to infection. To prevent infections:

- Help the person remember to wash their hands often with soap and water.

- Ask a health care provider about vaccines against the flu and pneumonia.

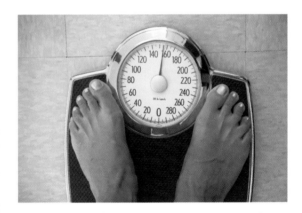

Tip: Track the person's weight daily. Weight gain of 2 or more pounds in a day and 5 or more pounds in a week can be a sign of a problem.

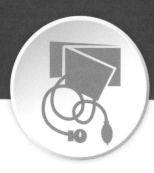

High Blood Pressure

Basic Facts

High blood pressure (or hypertension) is a very common problem that affects over half of older persons. It usually develops over many years and causes no noticeable symptoms. Despite this, untreated high blood pressure can lead to heart disease, kidney problems, stroke, and even the progression of dementia. More rarely, very high blood pressure, especially when accompanied by sudden symptoms, is an emergency.

What is considered "high" blood pressure depends on the person's age and health. Blood pressure can also change depending on the time of day, the person's mood, and physical activity. So, if the person you care for has measurements that are different than usual, but the person feels okay, check again throughout the day for several days. You may notice a pattern. For more on normal blood pressure ranges and on how to measure it at home, see page 140.

Signs of a Possible Emergency

Consider calling 911 or taking the person to an emergency department or health care provider office **SOON** if the person has any of these problems:

- passing out
- chest pain or trouble breathing at rest
- any new or worsening:
  - numbness or weakness of the face, arms, or legs (especially on one side of the body)
  - confusion, trouble speaking or slurring words, change in behavior
  - trouble seeing in one or both eyes
  - trouble walking, dizziness, loss of balance or coordination, or falls
- no new or worsening symptoms, but the person's blood pressure is over 220 systolic AND/OR over 120 diastolic multiple times, measured at least 30 minutes apart when the person is resting and calm. (See page 140 for more on blood pressure.)

Other Important Signs

Consider contacting a health care provider by phone and/or setting up a medical visit **within 1–3 days if you notice:**

- frequent or severe headaches
- a nosebleed that takes more than a few minutes to stop
- new or worsening confusion or a change in behavior
- no new or worsening symptoms, but the person's blood pressure is over 180 systolic (but below 220) AND/OR over 110 diastolic (but below 120) multiple times, measured at least 30 minutes apart when the person is resting and calm. (See page 140 for more on blood pressure.)

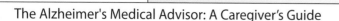

Tips on Providing Relief at Home

When possible, it's useful to have a way to measure blood pressure at home, especially if the person is on medication for high blood pressure. Blood pressure measurement includes two numbers. The higher number, called the systolic blood pressure, is a measurement of pressure when the heart is squeezing. The lower number, or diastolic blood pressure, is a measurement of pressure when the heart is relaxed. Experts disagree on the ideal blood pressure for older persons, including persons with dementia. Many consider a healthy reading to be a systolic reading under 140 and a diastolic reading under 90; however, recent guidelines encourage aiming for a systolic reading below 130 and a diastolic reading under 80.

If the person is being treated for high blood pressure:

- Follow any prescription medications, diet and exercise recommendations given by the health care provider.

- Measure and record the blood pressure frequently, as directed by the provider, so that you know the person's usual numbers. See page 140 for more on how to measure blood pressure.

- Ask the provider what range of blood pressure measurements is considered "high," as this varies from person to person.

- If you get a reading that is unusual, recheck again after 5 minutes, making sure the person is relaxed.

- Agitation or worry can make blood pressure rise. Help the person stay calm with relaxing music or an activity they enjoy. See page 30 for more on agitation.

If the person won't take their blood pressure medication:

- See Chapter 7 for tips on helping a person with dementia take medications.

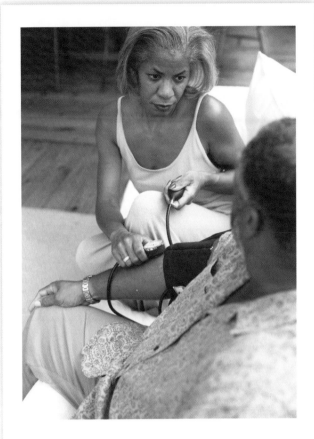

Tip: Measure and record the blood pressure frequently, as directed by the health care provider, so that you know the person's usual numbers.

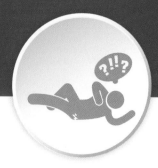

Hip Fracture

Basic Facts

A fractured (broken) hip is actually an injury to the thigh bone (femur) in the area close to the pelvis. Typically, the injury happens after a fall and is related to thin or weakened bones from osteoporosis. Most people with a hip fracture will have severe pain in the outer upper thigh or groin region, will not want to move the hip, and will be unable to stand or walk.

Treatment depends on where along the femur the fracture occurred. In most cases, the person will need surgery within 48 hours of the injury, followed by 2–6 weeks in a rehabilitation hospital and then another 3–4 weeks of in-home therapy.

Recovery can be very challenging, especially for someone with dementia. Aside from possible surgery complications, hospitalization can lead to more confusion or agitation than usual. The person may also have trouble following therapy directions. Despite these challenges, it's important to stick with the recovery program as much as possible so that the person can get back to doing what they could before the injury.

If the person fell and now has severe hip pain:

- Try to stay calm and call 911.
- Ask the person to stay where they are. Don't try to lift them. If they try to move, distract them with conversation or calm music.
- Place an ice pack covered in a towel on the painful area.
- Place a blanket over the person, and make them as comfortable as possible while waiting for help.

Signs of a Possible Emergency

Consider calling 911 or taking the person to an emergency department or health care provider office **SOON** if the person has any of these problems:

- **severe pain in the hip area** after a fall
- **inability to walk after a fall**
- after hip surgery:
  - **unbearable or increased hip pain;**
  - **chest pain or shortness of breath;**
  - **shaking chills;** or
  - **vital signs very different from usual,** especially rapid breathing or fever (see page 135 for how to measure vital signs)

Other Important Signs

Consider contacting a health care provider by phone and/or setting up a medical visit **within 1–3 days if a person has had hip surgery AND you notice:**

- the person **refuses treatments or physical therapies** at home
- **new or increased swelling** around surgery site
- **new or increased redness** around surgery site
- **new or increased pain or tenderness to the touch** around surgery site
- **new or increased drainage (fluid or bleeding) from the stitches,** especially if the drainage looks like thick, yellow pus
- **pain or swelling in the calf or leg**

Tips on Providing Relief at Home

Here are some care tips during recovery from a hip fracture:

If the person has pain:

- Talk to the health care provider about recommended pain medicines and the dosing schedule. Know their possible side effects and when to stop using them.

- If possible, use acetaminophen (Tylenol) instead of narcotic medications, as narcotics can cause increased confusion.

- To avoid constipation, ask the provider which laxatives to use with narcotic medications. Common recommendations are Senna along with plenty of fiber and fluids.

- To avoid periods without pain relief, give medicine on a regular schedule rather than first waiting for the pain to occur. It can take up to 2 hours for the person to feel the most relief after taking pain medicine.

- If the person is still having pain, talk to their provider, as there are a number of other non-drug pain relief options.

If the person is agitated or insists on walking on the operated leg:

- Try to stay calm and reassure them using gentle touch and eye contact.

- Avoid arguing with them about not walking. Tell them they need to rest to get better.

- Offer distractions like calm music or a snack. See page 30 for more on agitation.

- Try to figure out what they need. For example, look for signs of pain, hunger, or for needing to use the bathroom.

- If the problem is overwhelming, ask a health care provider or therapist for advice.

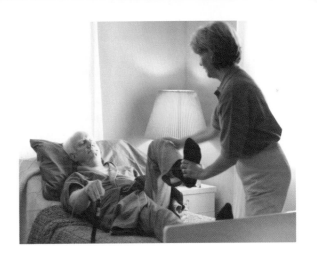

Taking Care of Your Own Safety and Stress

If the person is recovering from surgery and falls or slides to the floor:

- Call for help if you need it.

- Make sure it's safe to move them. If you think they may have a broken bone or neck injury, don't move them.

- If they can help themselves up, have them hold onto a sturdy object like a chair to pull up while you're there to steady them.

- If you must lift them, use your legs and not your back, keeping the person close to you.

If the person has had surgery and you're helping with rehabilitation exercises:

- Ask the physical therapist to show you ways to support the person safely without risking injury to yourself.

- Helping the person during the recovery period can be especially stressful. If needed, ask other family members or a provider for extra support so that you can take care of yourself.

See Chapter 3 for more ways to take care of yourself.

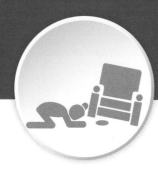

Hoarding

Basic Facts

A person who hoards collects things of little or no apparent value, often making their living space messy or unsafe. For example, a person with dementia may want to keep food in clothes drawers. Hoarding may be due to forgetfulness, boredom, or anxiety (like thinking someone may steal their things). Collecting or saving can also be something the person always did, but the habit becomes extreme as the dementia progresses. It can be tricky for a caregiver to help, as removing the items or even just tidying up can cause emotional upset.

Sudden hoarding habits, especially if they come with other sudden behavior or physical changes, could be a sign of delirium due to a new illness. But most of the time hoarding is a slowly developing problem that gets worse over time. As with other challenging behaviors, it's often best to focus on health or safety concerns while ignoring less urgent behaviors.

Signs of a Possible Emergency

Consider calling 911 or taking the person to an emergency department or health care provider office **SOON** if the person **is hoarding PLUS** has any of these problems:

- **signs of delirium**
  (see page 48 for more on delirium)

- **signs of dehydration**
  (see page 142 for more on dehydration)

- **vital signs very different from usual**, especially temperature over 101° F
  (see page 135 for how to measure vital signs)

Other Important Signs

Consider contacting a health care provider by phone and/or setting up a medical visit **within 1–3 days if you notice:**

- **sudden hoarding behaviors with signs of sickness** (like fever, cough, or weakness)

- **hoarding dangerous or unsafe objects** (such as jars containing urine, or moldy food)

If the person suddenly begins collecting or hiding things:

- Keep careful watch for signs that they're getting sick (like cough or abnormal vital signs), are in pain or have a physical need (like hunger).

- Problem solve using the tips on the following page.

- If the person is still not themselves after 24 hours, consider contacting the health care provider.

Tips on Providing Relief at Home

If the person has clutter and is upset by having it cleaned up:

- Focus on cleaning things that cause health or safety risks, and accept other clutter.

- Try removing hazards when the person isn't around.

- Take clutter away from the home (not in the garbage), because the person may try to bring it back into the home.

If the person has a cluttered living space and will accept some changes:

- Try putting clutter into bins and then see if they can decide which things to remove. Giving them a few items at a time to sort may help.

- Remove things at the person's pace. Avoid rushing them.

- Give them a good reason to remove things, such as sending the items to charities or family.

- Trade fresh food for spoiled or rotting food.

- Encourage them to reduce the number of each thing they collect. For example, ask them to save one newspaper at a time rather than a month of newspapers.

- Put labels on drawers to help them find things.

If the person hides and then loses things:

- Try to learn where the person tends to hide things and check these areas periodically.

- Check the wastebasket before emptying it.

- Put valuables (cash, jewelry, important papers) in a secure place.

- Have two copies of important things, such as glasses, keys, hearing aids, phones and remote control devices.

If the home is unsafe due to clutter, pets, bug problems or other issues:

- Focus on cleaning things that cause health or safety risks.

- Remove clutter close to hot things like radiators or stoves, and away from walking areas.

- Regularly check the pantry and refrigerator, and take out food that is spoiled or expired.

- Make sure the home has working smoke detectors and carbon monoxide detectors.

- Make sure that all utility bills are paid.

- Arrange to have needed repairs done and bug problems taken care of.

- For more ways to make the home safe and prevent falls, see page 68.

If the person is hoarding because they have untrue beliefs (like hiding food because someone is stealing it), see page 74 on delusions.

If the person gets angry or aggressive when you try cleaning up:

- Stay calm and reassuring.

- Remove or lock away any unsafe items (guns, knives, heavy items).

- Stop whatever you're doing that's upsetting them. You can try again later.

- Try to calm and distract them with another activity.

- If you can't calm them and it's safe to do so, give them space. Unless they're in immediate danger, restraining can make things worse.

- Get help if you need it.

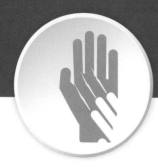

Basic Facts

Itching, scratching, and picking of the skin in older adults can have many causes. The most common causes are **dry skin, medications, bug bites,** and **fungal infections.** Many persons with dementia will repeat the same thing over and over, and this can happen with scratching even when the itch is minor. For this reason itching, picking and scratching can become a problem for some caregivers. **Dry skin** is the most common culprit. As we age it increases because our skin thins and is unable to hold moisture. Dry skin can be made worse by using harsh soaps, frequent bathing, bathing in hard water, or low humidity. Itchy skin with red bumps may be caused from **bug bites.**

- **Bedbugs** are small, oval, blood-feeding insects that live on furniture, beds, and in carpet. Their bites result in small flat or raised bumps that may be lined up in a row; itching can be severe.

- **Fleas** cause itchy, red bumps commonly found around the ankles, waist, armpits, and in the bends of knees and elbows. The red area often turns white when pressed. Fleas commonly infest pets and their environments, such as pet bedding and carpet.

- **Scabies** are microscopic parasites that burrow under the skin to live and lay eggs. They cause intense itching, especially at night, and a pimple-like rash. They commonly infest the wrist, underarm, elbow, between the fingers, waistline, buttocks, and groin area.

- If the person has been outside, itchy, red bumps may be caused by **mosquito** or **ant** bites.

Fungal infections can also cause itching. Common types include athlete's foot (a red, scaly rash on the feet and between the toes), ringworm (scaly patches on the skin with a raised border), and yeast (a bright red rash typically found in the armpits, under breasts, inner thighs, or private areas). (See page 108 for a photo of a yeast infection.)

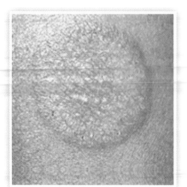

Ringworm

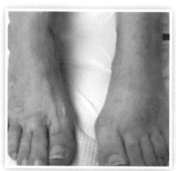

Athlete's foot

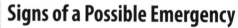

Signs of a Possible Emergency

Consider calling 911 or taking the person to an emergency department or health care provider office **SOON** if the person with itching skin has any of these problems:

- If the person has itching along with hives and difficulty breathing, or swelling of the lips or tongue, or fainting; this could indicate a severe allergic reaction

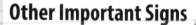

Other Important Signs

Consider contacting a health care provider by phone and/or setting up a medical visit **within 1–3 days** if the person has any of these problems:

- The person is causing harm to themselves by scratching and/or picking

- Signs of infection at the area the person is scratching or picking, such as marked redness, swelling, pus, increased pain, or fever

- Intense itching, especially at night, with red bumps and raised lines on the skin

- Rash lasting longer than 7 days

- Rash is painful and pain is increasing over time

- Fever with rash

Tips on Providing Relief at Home

- For dry skin, use moisturizing lotions daily, especially after bathing. Try lotions that are unscented and for sensitive skin, such as Cetaphil or Aveeno. Avoid drying soaps such as many deodorant soaps.

- If the person is incontinent, make sure they are clean and dry and use a skin protectant such as Vaseline or Desitin.

- For bites from bed bugs and fleas, obtain treatment for the problem. Relieve itching, swelling, and inflammation by applying cortisone cream and cold compresses.

- If you suspect bedbugs or fleas in your home, contact a pest control professional for ways to get rid of the problem.

- For scabies, contact a health care provider for treatment. Wash all clothing, bedding, and towels in hot soapy water and machine dry on high heat.

- For head or pubic lice, shave the affected area and/or use over-the-counter lice-killing shampoos or lotions. For body lice, help the person with personal hygiene and change clothes regularly. Wash all clothing, bedding, and towels in hot soapy water and machine dry on high heat. Check other people spending time in the home for lice.

- For a yeast infection, clean and dry the area twice a day, and leave open to air if possible. Apply an over-the-counter anti-fungal such as ketoconazole or clotrimazole.

- For athlete's foot or ringworm, apply an over-the-counter anti-fungal medicine such as butenafine or terbinafine. Keep affected feet dry.

- If the itching appears related to an allergy, stop using any items or products you suspect and watch for improvement.

- Trim nails short and cover itchy areas with a gauze bandage or long-sleeved shirt that is difficult to roll up and/or unbutton. You may also try having the person wear gloves, especially at night.

- If scratching or picking seems to be a habit related to dementia, in addition to treating possible causes (like dry skin), try getting them involved in activity or giving them something to do with their hands, such as a washcloth, busy blanket, or a small soft squeeze ball.

- For more information on rashes, see page 108.

If the person with itching has swollen lips and/or tongue, difficulty breathing or fainting:

- The person may be having an allergic reaction. The most common causes are foods, such as peanuts and shellfish, or medications.

- **Call 911 or get medical attention right away.**

If the person scratches and causes bleeding:

- Put pressure over the wound with gauze, a clean cloth, or a napkin until the bleeding stops.

- Gently clean the area with soap and water, apply pressure again if needed (because cleaning can re-start bleeding).

- Cover with a bandage to prevent further irritation at the site.

Taking Care of Your Own Safety and Stress

When helping apply medicines to rashes or providing wound care, always wear disposable gloves and wash your hands often.

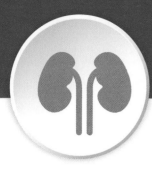

Kidney Disease

Basic Facts

The kidneys' main job is to remove waste, chemicals, and extra fluid from the body. They also release a chemical that helps the body make red blood cells, which carry oxygen throughout the body. Blood tests are used to test how well the kidneys are working.

When the kidneys don't work well, fluid and waste can build up in the body. This is called kidney disease or kidney failure. Because many medications are removed by the kidneys, a person with kidney disease may need to lower their medication dosage.

Common causes of kidney disease are uncontrolled diabetes and high blood pressure. Most kidney disease is chronic, because it doesn't get better; it stays the same or gets worse over time. A person with kidney disease may feel okay, especially if the disease is mild. As the disease progresses they may experience some or all of the following:

- Tiredness
- Muscle cramps at night
- Swelling of feet and legs
- Change in urination (either more or less)
- Lack of appetite
- Nausea and vomiting
- Dry and itchy skin
- Shortness of breath with activity
- Sleeping difficulties

If the kidney disease advances to where the kidneys are unable to remove waste or fluid from the blood, a decision may need to be made on whether to consider dialysis. If this happens, it's important to discuss the pros and cons of treatment options with your health care provider.

Signs of a Possible Emergency

Chronic kidney disease rarely causes an emergency; however, it can make the person more susceptible to heart failure or breathing problems; so, review those sections for more information.

Consider calling 911 or taking the person to an emergency department or health care provider office **SOON** if the person with kidney disease has any of these problems:

- **Heart beat is over 120 beats per minute or under 45 beats per minute,** especially if the person feels weak or dizzy or has chest pain
- **Markedly decreased or no urine** for 12 hours or more
- Any new or severely worsening problem with **breathing**, the **heart**, or **energy level**

Other Important Signs

Consider contacting a health care provider by phone and/or setting up a medical visit **within 1–3 days if you notice any of the following in the person with kidney disease:**

- Feeling tired
- Muscle cramps at night
- Swelling of feet and legs
- Urinating more or urinating less
- Lack of appetite
- Nausea and vomiting
- Dry and itchy skin
- Feeling short of breath
- Sleeping difficulties

Tips on Providing Relief at Home

There are many things you can do to manage kidney disease at home:

- Keep track of the person's weight daily. A sudden increase in weight of more than 2–3 pounds may mean that the person is holding onto fluid and needs medical attention.

- Help the person maintain a healthy lifestyle by exercising, avoiding smoking and alcohol use, and getting rest.

- Remind the person to take their medications as prescribed.

- Consult with a nutritionist for a diet plan that includes low amounts of salt (for example, by avoiding foods like deli meats, soy sauce and frozen foods), potassium and protein.

- Avoid star fruit. This fruit contains a toxin that can cause seizures, confusion, or other serious problems in persons with advanced kidney disease.

If the person becomes short of breath when doing everyday activities:

- Take breaks often. For example, when helping someone get dressed, encourage rest after putting on each piece of clothing.

- Use assistive devices. For example, use a shower chair.

- Help the person to use the bathroom regularly to avoid having to rush to the bathroom.

- Place chairs throughout the home to allow the person to stop and catch their breath while walking.

Treatment for kidney disease involves:

- Treating the cause; for example diabetes or high blood pressure.

- Diet. The person should work with a nutritionist to follow a diet low in sodium and protein.

- Caution with medication. When a prescription is new or changed, always ask the health care provider if it needs to be adjusted because of the person's kidneys.

- Regular medical follow-up. In mild disease, this usually means the person's primary care provider. In more advanced disease, regular consultation with a kidney specialist is usually advisable.

Preventing Infections

People with kidney disease are more susceptible to infection. To prevent infections:

- Help the person remember to wash their hands often with soap and water.

- Ask a health care provider about vaccines against the flu and pneumonia.

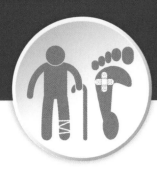

Leg and Foot Wounds

Basic Facts

Due to aging and chronic illness, many older persons have poor blood flow and/or swelling of their lower legs and feet. This can lead to lower leg wounds (or ulcers) that are slow to heal or keep coming back. Even minor injuries can cause serious problems if not carefully watched and treated.

There are four main types of leg and foot ulcers:

- **Venous ulcers:** Leaking valves in the leg veins can lead to swelling, varicose or spider veins, and ulcers. The ulcers are typically found near the inside of the ankle; they may weep clear fluid.

- **Arterial ulcers:** These ulcers are often found in people with poor blood flow in their arteries. They commonly form over bony areas of the toes and tend to look circular or "punched out."

- **Diabetic (neuropathic) ulcers:** These are typically found on the bottom of the foot in persons with diabetes.

- **Pressure ulcers:** These are caused from sitting or lying in the same position for too long. (See page 106 for more on pressure ulcers.)

In all cases, daily attention to the skin with early treatment of any problems is important to prevent infection and the possibility of losing a part of the foot or leg.

Signs of a Possible Emergency

Consider calling 911 or taking the person to an emergency department or health care provider office **SOON** if the person has any of these problems:

- a toe that turns black
- something sharp gets stuck in the foot
- a wound bleeds and doesn't stop after 15–30 minutes
- a wound has a large, growing area of redness around it or red streaks coming from it
- shaking chills, especially if accompanied by fever
- vital signs very different from usual, especially temperature over 100° F (see page 135 for how to measure vital signs)

Other Important Signs

Consider contacting a health care provider by phone and/or setting up a medical visit **within 1–3 days** if the person has had any of these problems:

- changes in a wound that suggest infection:
  - new or increased swelling, redness or warmth around a wound
  - increased wound size
  - new or increased pain or tenderness to the touch
  - new or increased fluid from the wound, especially if it looks like thick, yellow pus
  - new or increased foul smell from a wound
- a wound that isn't improving after 10 days
- any new break in the skin (cracked, scaly, blistered, red skin)
- skin areas that stay rough, red or painful (this can be an early sign of a developing wound)

Tips on Providing Relief at Home

If the person you care for develops a leg or foot wound:

- See their medical provider for specific wound care advice, including recommendations for bandages or wraps that may speed healing.

- Clean the affected area daily with a mild soap and saline or warm water.

- If the wound is open, apply a layer of petroleum jelly or antibiotic ointment over the wound.

- Cover the wound with a non-stick bandage like Telfa. Try to avoid putting tape directly on the skin by wrapping the area with dry gauze or an Ace bandage.

- For pain relief, use acetaminophen (Tylenol) or another pain medication recommended by their provider. Don't give aspirin, BC, or Goody powders as these can make bleeding worse.

- Relieve pressure on the affected area by encouraging movement, helping the person shift positions, and placing padding where needed. Ask a provider about special support cushions.

- If you have a smartphone, take photos of the area to show or send to the health care provider.

If the person has venous ulcer(s) with leg swelling:

- Raise the legs above heart level for 30 minutes 3-4 times a day (or whenever they're at rest).

- See page 94 for more on lower leg swelling.

If the person has arterial ulcer(s):

- Help the person to sit with legs dangling to increase blood flow.

- Raise the head of the bed 5-8 inches. This will increase blood flow to the legs at night while the person sleeps.

- Watch the feet carefully. Get medical help right away if you notice these signs of blocked blood flow: severe pain, coolness to the touch or color change (blue or pale) in one leg or foot.

If the person has diabetic foot ulcer(s):

- After bathing, dry the feet and apply a thin coat of petroleum jelly or unscented skin cream to all areas except between the toes.

- See the health care provider for specific advice on footwear and bandages.

Things you can do to prevent leg and foot wounds:

- Encourage the person to eat a healthy diet, be physically active, and not smoke. If possible, have them walk every day to keep blood flowing.

- Encourage the person to always wear shoes or slippers and long pants or knee high socks except when bathing or in bed.

- Check the skin daily for red areas, cracks or sores, and treat problem areas early.

- Clean the skin daily with a mild soap and apply moisturizer to areas without wounds.

Taking Care of Your Own Safety and Stress

Wear disposable gloves and wash your hands thoroughly before and after cleaning a wound or changing bandages.

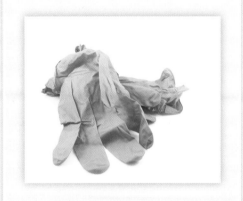

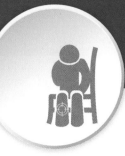

Leg Swelling

Basic Facts

Lower leg swelling is common in older persons, often developing over months to years. This chronic swelling is due to poor circulation, extra fluid in the body, or both, and is usually not an emergency. Leaky leg veins, being overweight, taking certain medications, standing or sitting for long periods, and high salt diets can make swelling worse. Chronic leg swelling can also be a complication of many illnesses, including heart, liver, lung or kidney disease, and even sleep apnea.

Lower leg swelling that develops over hours to days can be more urgent. Sometimes, the sudden swelling is just the worsening of a chronic problem. However, it can also be a sign of something new and more serious, like a blood clot, skin infection, or injury, especially if the swelling is in only one leg. For this reason, a health care provider should be contacted about any new or worsening lower leg swelling.

Signs of a Possible Emergency

Consider calling 911 or taking the person to an emergency department or health care provider office **SOON** if the person has any of these problems:

- sudden or worsening lower leg(s) swelling along with **severe trouble breathing and/or chest pain, tightness or pressure**
- **toes that have turned cold and either white or blue,** which could mean blocked blood flow
- leg swelling that **develops rapidly after a fall or injury**
- sudden lower leg(s) swelling with **vital signs very different from usual,** such as fast breathing, fast pulse, low blood pressure or fever (see page 135 for how to measure vital signs)

Other Important Signs

Consider contacting a health care provider by phone and/or setting up a medical visit **within 1–3 days if you notice:**

- **tenderness, warmth and/or redness in swollen leg area**
- **new or worsening leg swelling in a person who has heart, kidney, lung or liver disease,** without any of the urgent symptoms listed above
- **a leg wound or ulcer that has signs of infection** including:
  - wound is getting bigger
  - worsening redness
  - swelling or pain around the wound
  - new or worsening drainage or pus from the wound
- **new shortness of breath,** especially with everyday activities
- lower leg swelling and pain that happens **after a fall or injury**
- **any new leg or body swelling** without other symptoms
- **lower leg swelling that doesn't get better** after doing home care tips

Tips on Providing Relief at Home

If the person has chronic lower leg swelling, here are some tips for managing the problem at home:

- Raise the legs above heart level for 30 minutes 3-4 times a day (ideally whenever at rest).

- Encourage leg movement, such as walking, every day. If a person sits a lot, ask them to move their feet up and down at the ankle throughout the day.

- Use compression leg stockings found at most drug stores (ask the health care provider if a prescription strength is needed). For persons who are unable to wear support stockings, an IPC (intermittent pneumatic compression) pump may be recommended.

- Take good care of the skin and watch carefully for cracks or sores.

  - Clean the legs with a mild soap and apply moisturizer every day.

  - If itching is a problem, keep the person's nails short and ask the health care provider about a soothing prescription steroid cream.

- Offer a healthy diet low in salt. Help the person avoid smoking and keep a healthy weight.

- Ask a provider to review the person's medications to see if any might cause or aggravate swelling.

- Help the person to manage other chronic medical problems that can worsen swelling.

- If the person develops a sore on the leg or foot:

  - See a provider or wound specialist

  - Use compression bandages to speed healing

  - Watch for signs of infection

  - If you have a smartphone, take photos of the area to show or send to the health care provider.

What to Watch Out For

- **Skin changes and infection:** Long periods of leg swelling can cause skin to become dry, itchy, discolored, and weeping with fluid. Open sores ("ulcers") can appear and get infected. Follow the skin care tips on this page and watch for these signs of infection:

  - Fever/chills

  - New or increasing swelling, redness, pain, or warmth, especially if accompanied by (often mild) fever

  - Pus draining from a sore

- **Blood clot in the leg:** Poor circulation can lead to a blood clot in the leg. Bring the person to a health care provider if they develop a bright red, warm, swollen, painful area, especially if only in one leg.

- **Blood clot in the lung:** Blood clot(s) in the leg can travel to the lung. This is an emergency. Watch for:

  - Sudden shortness of breath

  - Sharp chest pain

  - Coughing up blood

  - Fast heart rate

Taking Care of Your Own Safety and Stress

- Wash your hands thoroughly before and after cleaning a wound or changing bandages and, if possible, wear disposable gloves.

See Chapter 3 for more ways to take care of yourself.

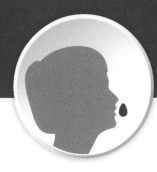

Nosebleeds

Basic Facts

Most nosebleeds aren't serious and can be stopped at home. Blood vessels in the front of the nose are close to the surface and can be easily irritated by dry air, a virus, allergies, or cigarette smoke. These blood vessels can also be damaged from picking or injury to the nose.

Occasionally, a nosebleed can be heavy and hard to stop. Other times, the person may have frequent smaller nosebleeds despite good home care. In these cases, medical treatment may be necessary.

If the person's nose is bleeding:

- Try to stay calm and reassure them that you can help.
- Help the person sit up comfortably.
- Ask them to lean a bit forward at the waist so they don't swallow blood.
- Using tissues, apply steady pressure to the soft part of the nostrils for 15 minutes ("pinching" the nose closed).
- If possible, place an ice pack wrapped in a towel on the bony part of the nose while pinching nostrils.
- After 15 minutes, release pressure. If bleeding continues, pinch nostrils for another 15 minutes.
- If bleeding continues after holding pressure for a total of 30 minutes, consider getting medical care right away.

Signs of a Possible Emergency

Consider calling 911 or taking the person to an emergency department or health care provider office **SOON** if the person has a **nosebleed AND** any of these problems:

- **passing out**
- **chest pain**
- **new dizziness, weakness or confusion**
- **trouble staying awake**
- **nose injury** or recent **nose surgery**
- a **nose tumor**
- **bleeding that is heavy and/or will not stop** after trying home care, especially if the person takes a blood thinning medicine or has a blood clotting disorder
- **vital signs very different from usual** (see page 135 for how to measure vital signs)

Other Important Signs

Consider contacting a health care provider by phone and/or setting up a medical visit **within 1–3 days if you notice:**

- **frequent nosebleeds,** even if you can stop them, especially if the person is on a blood thinning medicine
- **easy bleeding in other areas,** including skin bruising

Tips on Providing Relief at Home

If the person is very upset by a nosebleed:

- Try to stay calm and reassuring.

- Offer a distraction like music, singing or television as you help.

- If the sight of blood upsets them, cover their clothes with a towel.

- Give simple one-step directions. You may need to show the person how to pinch the nostrils, or you may need to hold the pressure yourself.

- If the person is still upset or agitated and you can't safely stop the bleeding, give the person space and call for help.

If the person gets nosebleeds often:

- Dry air may be a cause, so use an air humidifier in the bedroom where the person sleeps.

- Keep the inside of the nose moist by applying a thin layer of petroleum jelly (Vaseline) to the inside of the nostrils twice a day.

- If the person is picking at or blowing their nose often, keep their nails short and try to distract them with something they like to do.

- Avoid exposure to cigarette smoke, dust, pet dander, or other air irritants.

- Talk to a health care provider about medicines the person takes, like nose sprays or blood thinners, that may be causing the bleeding.

What to Watch Out For

- **Nausea or vomiting:** Swallowing blood can cause an upset stomach.

To prevent this, ask the person to sit up and lean forward so that blood drips out of the nose rather than down the throat.

Taking Care of Your Own Safety and Stress

- Keep disposable gloves handy and wear them while helping with a nosebleed.

See Chapter 3 for more ways to take care of yourself.

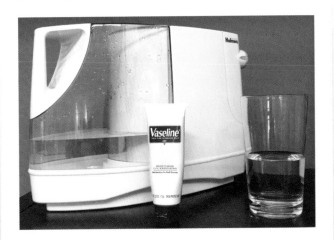

Tip: Keep the inside of the nose moist. Use an air humidifier in the bedroom where the person sleeps and apply Vaseline to the inside of the nostrils twice a day.

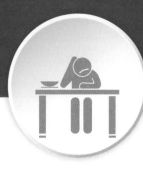

Not Eating or Drinking

Basic Facts

Saying "no" to food or drink is common in people with dementia. Slowly losing the ability to feel hunger and thirst is a natural part of late stage dementia.

When not eating or drinking happens more suddenly, over days to weeks, it may not just be the dementia getting worse. Here are some possible causes:

- **New or worsening illness.** A cold, urine infection, stomach problem, worsening chronic illness, or even constipation can make a person with dementia eat or drink less.

- **Sad or worried mood.** Feeling sad or worried can take away appetite.

- **Pain.** Problems with the teeth and gums, or pain anywhere else, can take away appetite.

- **Medications.** Side effects of many medicines take away the appetite or bother the stomach.

- **Problems with where or how food is offered.** Any change in where they're eating, what they're offered to eat, and who is helping them can affect appetite.

With some trouble-shooting, caregivers can often get the person eating and drinking again.

Signs of a Possible Emergency

Consider calling 911 or taking the person to an emergency department or health care provider office **SOON** if the person has any of these problems:

- **severe belly pain or belly pain that gets worse over time,** especially with **vomiting or fever**

- belly is **swollen**, **hard** or **very tender** to the touch

- **signs of dehydration** (see page 142 for more on dehydration)

- **signs of delirium** (see page 48 for more on delirium)

- **vital signs very different from usual,** especially temperature above 101° F (see page 135 for how to measure vital signs)

Other Important Signs

Consider contacting a health care provider by phone and/or setting up a medical visit **within 1–3 days if the person is having problems eating or drinking AND you notice:**

- **suddenly not eating or drinking for 24 hours,** even without any new signs of illness

- **no bowel movement for 4 days**

- the problem started after taking a new medication

- faster than usual breathing rate

- **low grade fever for longer than 24 hours** (see page 70 for more on fever)

- any other sign that makes you think the person is getting sick or that worries you

Tips on Providing Relief at Home

Here are some things you can try at home when the person is not eating or drinking well and you don't think the problem is from a new or worsening illness, medication, or pain (for those problems, talk with the health care provider):

- Offer food at the same times each day.

- Try offering a larger breakfast, as this is when people are often hungriest.

- Offer foods and drinks that the person likes, and try new things. A person with dementia may have changes in taste. For fluids, try flavored water, popsicles, or milkshakes.

- Make sure the food and drink are at a temperature the person enjoys.

- Make eating and drinking easier by cutting up food, offering easy-to-swallow foods, using a white plate (so food is easier to see), and giving just one utensil.

- Make sure meals and snacks aren't rushed. Keep noises low and TV off. Try playing calm music and eating together.

- Encourage the person to be active to help the appetite.

- For more information on nutrition and weight including nutrition at the end of life, see pages 144-145.

- See page 46 if you think the person has chewing and/or swallowing problems.

- Check the mouth for sores, redness or bad teeth. See page 56 if you think the person has tooth problems.

- See page 58 if the person seems sad or worried most of the time.

What to Watch Out For

- **Low fluid in the body (dehydration):** A person with dementia can quickly become dehydrated. Some signs of dehydration are:

  - Dry mouth and tongue
  - Urinating very little
  - Fast heart beat
  - Slow, weak, or low energy

If you've tried the tips on this page but the person still seems dehydrated, get medical help.

- **Weight loss:** Weight loss happens when the person is not getting enough calories. In addition to the tips on this page:

  - Take the person to the health care provider to be checked, especially if they've lost more than 5 pounds in a week or 10 pounds in 1–3 months.

  - Offer high calorie high-fat foods, like butter and milkshakes. Talk to a nutritionist for ideas.

Taking Care of Your Own Safety and Stress

When helping a person who is not eating or drinking:

- Never put your hand or fingers between teeth.

- Keep sharp utensils, like knives, off the table. Give plastic utensils if they get upset during meals, and never force a person to eat. You can try again later.

See Chapter 3 for more ways to take care of yourself.

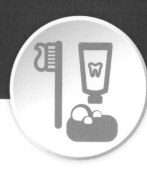

Basic Facts

In early or mid-stage dementia, caregivers may have concerns about the person's ability to keep up with their personal and home care. These concerns are especially worrisome if the person's health or safety is at risk. For example, the person may forget to bathe or wash their clothes, stop taking their medicine, or keep their home so cluttered that it's hard to walk.

If the changes are sudden, especially if they come with other symptoms, the person may be getting sick. If the problems come on slowly, they're more likely due to forgetting, being physically unable to do the activities, or depression. Or possibly the person doesn't find personal or home care important and will be upset by your attempts to help. If this happens, decide which concerns are most important and be creative in problem solving.

Signs of a Possible Emergency

Consider calling 911 or taking the person to an emergency department or health care provider office **SOON** if the person has any of these problems:

- signs of delirium
  (see page 48 for more on delirium)

- signs of dehydration
  (see page 142 for more on dehydration)

- vital signs very different from usual, especially temperature over 101° F (see page 135 for how to measure vital signs)

Other Important Signs

Consider contacting a health care provider by phone and/or setting up a medical visit **within 1–3 days if you notice:**

- not taking care of oneself with signs of sickness (like fever, cough, or diarrhea)

- not taking care of oneself along with other sudden behavior changes (like sleepiness or weakness)

- unplanned weight loss

- skin sores or rashes

If the person gets angry or aggressive when you try to help:

- Stay calm and reassuring.

- Remove or lock away any unsafe items (guns, knives, heavy items).

- Stop whatever you're doing that's upsetting them. You can try again later.

- Try to distract them with another activity.

- If you can't calm them and it's safe to do so, give them space. Unless they're in immediate danger, restraining them can make things worse.

- Get help if you need it.

Tips on Providing Relief at Home

A person with a sudden change in their ability to take care of themselves should be watched carefully for signs of new illness, pain, depression, or a physical need. If you are concerned, have them assessed by a health care provider. If these are not the cause, focus on helping with personal or home care activities that are a health or safety risk.

If the person isn't keeping clean:

- Try simply reminding the person about changing clothes, bathing, teeth brushing, hair and nail care. If needed, offer to help with the activities.

- Keep out only the clothes that are appropriate for the weather.

- Treat any skin sores or injuries (see page 114).

- If they refuse or are upset by your help, see resisting care (see page 110).

If the person isn't taking care of their medical conditions:

- Help with medications by giving the medicine yourself, giving reminders or using pillboxes. For more on managing medications, see Chapter 7.

- If they're on a special diet, keep proper food in the house.

- If you're still concerned, talk with a health care provider.

If the person suddenly isn't taking care of themselves:

- Keep careful watch for signs that they're getting sick (like cough or abnormal vital signs), are in pain, depressed, or have a physical need (like hunger).

- Try the tips above to problem solve.

- If the person is still not themselves after 24 hours, consider contacting the health care provider.

If the home is unsafe due to clutter, pets, bug problems or other issues:

- Focus on cleaning things that cause health or safety risks.

- Remove clutter close to hot things like radiators or stoves, and away from walking areas. If they're upset when you remove items, see page 86 on hoarding.

- Regularly check the pantry and refrigerator, and dispose of food that is spoiled or expired.

- Make sure the home has working smoke detectors and carbon monoxide detectors.

- Make sure that all bills are paid.

- Arrange to have needed repairs done and bug problems taken care of.

- For more ways to make the home safe and prevent falls, see page 68.

- If the person isn't eating or drinking well, see page 98.

- If the person has signs of depression, including seeming sad or tearful most of the time, see page 58.

- If you're still concerned, consider a hired aide or change in living situation.

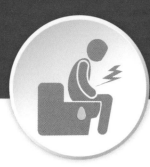

Pain with Urination

Basic Facts

Pain, discomfort or "burning" with urination can be a sign of bladder or kidney infection (a urinary tract infection/UTI). This is especially true if the pain comes along with fever, blood in the urine, or pain in the lower belly or back. Other causes include skin irritation in the private area, injury from a bladder catheter or from repeated touching, and prostate problems in men. More rarely, pain can be from a blockage in the urinary system, a sexually transmitted disease, or a medication side effect. In most cases, painful urination is not an emergency and can be managed at home.

Signs of a Possible Emergency

Consider calling 911 or taking the person to an emergency department or health care provider office **SOON** if the person has any of these problems:

- **shaking chills**
- **severe lower belly or lower back pain** (the person is doubled over, crying, or can't move)
- **blood clots** in the urine
- the person **can't urinate** (except for small amounts), despite feeling like they have to
- **signs of delirium** (see page 48 for more on delirium)
- **symptoms lasting longer than 7 days**
- **vital signs very different from usual,** especially temperature above 101° F (see page 135 for how to measure vital signs)

Other Important Signs

Consider contacting a health care provider by phone and/or setting up a medical visit **within 1–3 days if you notice:**

- **Temperature above 99° F** or 1.2° F above the person's normal body temperature (see page 70 for more on fever) and/or **lower belly or lower back pain** or **painful urination**
- **blood in the urine**
- **pus or fluid** from the vagina or penis
- **sudden changes in urinary habits** (new or worse urine accidents, going to the bathroom more often) without any other cause and lasting for more than 4 days

Tips on Providing Relief at Home

If the person has pain with urination:

- Offer at least 6 cups of fluid each day.

- Offer acetaminophen (Tylenol) or another pain reliever recommended by a health care provider. The medicine phenazopyridine (Pyridium) is also available over-the-counter to help relieve painful urination. (This medicine will turn the urine orange or reddish.)

- If the person is being treated for a urinary tract infection (UTI), give medicines as directed.

If the person is having trouble "going"/urinating (urine retention):

- Give privacy and plenty of time in the bathroom.

- Turn on the faucet, place the person's hands in warm water, or run warm water over the private area while they try to urinate.

- Encourage them to lean forward and/or gently push on their belly while on the toilet.

- Get medical help right away if they've gotten little or no urine out after 8 hours, especially if they also have worsening lower belly pain.

If the person has vaginal dryness or irritation:

- Wash the outside of the vagina with unscented soap and water and dry it well once a day to clean any urine leakage. Avoid bubble baths and douches, and wipe from front to back.

- Encourage the person to wear loose fitting clothes and cotton underwear.

- For dryness, talk with a health care provider about vaginal creams and tablets. Vaginal moisturizers such as Replens® or Lubrin® can also help and are available over-the-counter.

If the person is rubbing or scratching the private area:

- Check them for rash or skin problems. Treat mild skin irritation with things like A&D ointment, over-the-counter hydrocortisone cream, zinc oxide paste, or Vaseline. See a health care provider if it's severe or doesn't get better in a few days.

- Gently remind them to not touch the area, and offer a distraction. Give them something else to do with their hands. See page 30 for more tips on agitation.

What to Watch Out For

- **Urinary Tract Infection:** Pain with urination can be a sign of a bladder or kidney infection. (See page 124) Tell a health care provider if you also notice these signs:

  - Fever

  - Blood in the urine

  - Pain in the lower belly or back (Press down on the lower belly and tap the lower back to check for this.)

  - Changes in urinary habits (new or more accidents, going more often)

Taking Care of Your Own Safety and Stress

For your protection, wear disposable gloves when helping with personal care.

See Chapter 3 for more ways to take care of yourself.

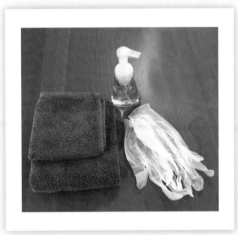

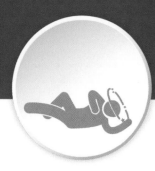

Passing Out

Basic Facts

When a person passes out (faints, blacks out, falls out), it's usually because they've had a sudden drop in blood flow to the brain. The person may feel suddenly weak or dizzy, then fall and be unable to respond for a minute or so, until they "come to" (awaken, become conscious) on their own. This happens most often when an older person stands up, since the shift in position can temporarily reduce blood flow to the brain. Medications, dehydration, viral illnesses, alcohol, being overheated, feeling pain or worry, having just gone to the bathroom, and eating a heavy meal can all lower blood pressure and make passing out more likely.

Passing out in older persons can be serious, either because the problem that caused it is serious (for example, a new heart problem) or because the person fell and became injured. It's often not obvious what caused a passing out spell, so most people should see a health care provider when it occurs.

Signs of a Possible Emergency

Consider calling 911 or taking the person to an emergency department or health care provider office **SOON** if the person has any of these problems:

- passing out with **no breathing, no pulse, or the person doesn't "come to" within 60 seconds**

- passing out after being **physically active**, or after having **severe chest pain, tightness, shortness of breath, or a lot of bleeding**

- the person isn't back to themselves after "coming to":

  - **new symptoms** like **confusion, trouble moving a body part or not walking normally**

  - **seizure** before, during, or after passing out

  - **serious injury** (like a possible broken bone)

  - **vomiting** more than once after hitting head

- passing out in a **diabetic with low blood sugar**

- **signs of dehydration** (see page 142 for more on dehydration)

- **vital signs very different from usual** (see page 135 for how to measure vital signs)

Other Important Signs

Consider contacting a health care provider by phone and/or setting up a medical visit **within 1–3 days if you notice:**

- any passing out (even without urgent signs)

Tips on Providing Relief at Home

In most cases, you'll need to act fast after a person falls or passes out. But, sometimes the person will feel differently right before passing out—they might feel dizzy, weak, shaky, or have "tunnel vision"— giving you the chance to prevent an episode.

If the person says they feel like they might pass out or gets suddenly unsteady:

- Help them to lie down and raise their legs about 12 inches above their heart level. Try a recliner or propping the legs up with pillows on the couch.

- If they can't lie down, help them to sit and put their head between their legs.

- Loosen any tight clothing.

- If the person has diabetes and you think they might have low blood sugar, give them a food or drink with sugar in it (like juice) and check their blood sugar.

- If possible, check pulse, breathing rate and blood pressure.

- If the person has vital signs different from usual, doesn't feel back to normal within a few minutes, or has any other symptoms, consider getting medical care right away.

Here are some general things you can do to prevent passing out:

- Offer at least 6 cups of fluid each day to prevent dehydration.

- For those who feel faint when going from "down" (sitting or lying) to "up," always keep something sturdy nearby to help them be steady. Gently remind them to change positions slowly.

- If the person feels faint after big meals, try offering smaller snacks throughout the day.

- If the person has low blood pressure, ask the health care provider about adding more salt to the diet.

- For some, special leg stockings can help with circulation.

- Ask a pharmacist or health care provider to review the person's medications for possible effects on blood pressure.

What to Watch Out For

- **A fall associated with passing out.** Check for serious injuries before helping them up. See page 68 for more on what to do right after a fall.

- **Confusion or weakness:** Right after a fall, the person may seem stunned. After a few minutes, they should seem more like themselves. If they don't, contact a health care provider.

- **Head injury:** See page 76 for what to do if you think the person hit their head.

- **Minor scrapes and cuts:** Older skin can tear easily. See page 114 for more on caring for minor skin injuries.

If the person passes out and falls (or falls and then passes out):

Try to stay calm. Most people wake up soon. **Call 911** and while waiting for them to arrive:

- Check for breathing and pulse.

- If there's no breathing or no pulse, and resuscitation is part of the care plan, start CPR (cardiopulmonary resuscitation). To learn CPR, call the American Heart Association at 1-877-242-4277 or visit www.cpr.heart.org.

- If they're breathing and have a pulse:
  - lie them on their side to prevent choking
  - loosen tight clothes
  - put pressure on any bleeding
  - for diabetics with low blood sugar, place sugar inside cheek
  - cover them with a blanket if it's cold
  - after they "come to," see page 68 for tips on how to check for injuries

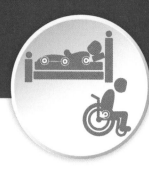

Pressure Ulcers

Basic Facts

A pressure ulcer (pressure sore or bed sore) is a wound caused by lying or sitting too long in the same position. Pressure between a bone (like the elbow, tailbone, hip or heel) and the surface below pinches the tissue in between, keeping blood from flowing and causing damage. This can happen in a few short hours if someone can't shift their weight, so it's very important to help people change position often to prevent skin breakdown. Once an ulcer develops, it can be slow to heal.

Aside from lack of movement, ulcers can also occur when fragile skin rubs against surfaces or fabrics (such as when a person slides down bed sheets), when skin is left moist or unclean (such as after urine accidents) or when the person isn't eating or drinking well. Because all of these situations are common in later stages of dementia, careful attention to skin is vital for ulcer prevention and healing.

Signs of a Possible Emergency

Consider calling 911 or taking the person to an emergency department or health care provider office **SOON** if the person has any of these problems:

- **shaking chills**
- **vital signs very different from usual,** especially temperature over 101° F (see page 135 for how to measure vital signs)

Other Important Signs

Consider contacting a health care provider by phone and/or setting up a medical visit **within 1–3 days if you notice:**

- **a change in a wound that may suggest infection** (see box at left)
- **any new break in the skin** (cracked, scaly, blistered, red skin)
- **any skin areas that stay rough, red or painful** especially over bony areas (this can be an early sign of an ulcer)
- **any new rash or hives**
- **any skin area that is painful and doesn't get better with acetaminophen** (Tylenol)

What to Watch Out For

- **Signs of a wound infection:**
  - new or increased swelling
  - new or increased redness
  - increased wound size
  - new or increased pain or tenderness to the touch
  - new or increased drainage (fluid) from the wound, especially if the drainage looks like thick, yellow pus

Tips on Providing Relief at Home

Here are some things you can do to prevent pressure ulcers:

- Take good care of the skin and check carefully for red areas, cracks or sores.

  - Clean skin with a mild soap and apply moisturizer every day.

  - If the person has urine or bowel accidents, keep the area as clean and dry as possible and use a moisture barrier (such as A&D ointment or Desitin cream).

- Offer at least 6 cups of fluid each day and encourage a healthy diet high in protein (such as fish, poultry and nuts).

- Encourage the person to move as much as they can. If movement is limited:

  - While in a chair, ask them to shift positions every 10 minutes or help them to change their hip and tailbone position every 30 minutes.

  - While in bed, turn the person every 2 hours to relieve pressure points.

- Prevent skin shearing injuries when helping move the person in bed. Whenever possible, help the person to lift rather than slide across sheets, or use a draw sheet. Keep sheets clean, dry and wrinkle-free.

If a pressure ulcer develops:

- Get medical attention right away.

- Relieve pressure on the affected area by encouraging movement, helping the person shift positions, and placing padding where needed. Ask a provider about special support cushions.

- Offer at least 6 cups of fluid each day and encourage a healthy diet high in protein (fish, lean meats, nuts), vitamin C (citrus, spinach), vitamin A (leafy greens, yellow squash) and zinc (red meat, seafood).

- Use acetaminophen (Tylenol) to relieve pain. Avoid ibuprofen or aspirin, as these can lead to bleeding. If the person still has pain after taking medication, talk to the health care provider.

- Watch for warning signs of infection. (See box on previous page.)

- If you have a smartphone, take photos of the area to show or send to the health care provider.

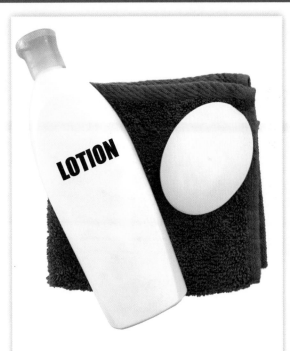

Tip: Clean the skin with a mild soap and apply moisturizer every day.

Taking Care of Your Own Safety and Stress

- Wash your hands thoroughly before and after cleaning a wound or changing bandages and, if possible, wear disposable gloves.

See Chapter 3 for more ways to take care of yourself.

Rash

Basic Facts

Rashes are changes to the color or surface of the skin and can be caused by many different things. Most rashes are not a serious problem and can be treated at home. Some common causes of rash include:

- **Contact dermatitis:** Itchy bumps or blisters, sometimes with fluid oozing out, caused by skin contact with an irritant or allergen. Common causes include cosmetics; jewelry containing leather, nickel, or cobalt; rubber or latex; antibiotic ointments; and urine and/or stool. Plants such as poison ivy, oak, or sumac can also cause this rash.

- **Stasis dermatitis:** This rash occurs over the lower legs in people whose legs are swollen much or all of the time. The skin is usually red or brown, itchy and can become flaky.

- **Yeast infection:** Bright red, itchy areas where the skin tends to stay moist (armpits, skin folds, groin). Poor hygiene and taking antibiotics can make this rash worse.

- **Shingles:** This painful red rash with fluid-filled blisters usually occurs in a line on one side of the body or face. It's caused by a virus and may come with symptoms like fever or headache.

- **Hives:** Itchy red bumps caused by an allergic reaction and that often resemble mosquito bites. They can occur anywhere on the body, but are often prominent in waistband areas. Medications, foods and insect stings are some common causes of hives. Hives can be an emergency if the person also has swelling around the mouth or trouble breathing.

If the person you care for develops a rash without any warning signs of more serious illness, think about what might be causing the problem and use the home care tips for treatment and prevention.

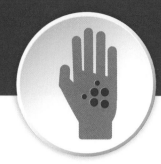

Contact dermatitis from allergy to a sheepskin bootie.

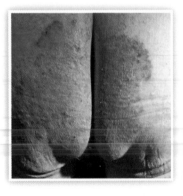

Yeast infection from moisture.

Signs of a Possible Emergency

Consider calling 911 or taking the person to an emergency department or health care provider office **SOON** if the person has any of these problems:

- **rash with difficulty breathing, swelling of the lips or tongue, or passing out**
- **vital signs very different from usual,** especially temperature above 101° F (see page 135 for how to measure vital signs)

Other Important Signs

Consider contacting a health care provider by phone and/or setting up a medical visit **within 1–3 days** if the person has any of these problems:

- rash with low grade fever
- rash that lasts longer than 7 days
- an area of skin that's bright red and warm to the touch, swollen and tender
- painful red rash with blisters in a line pattern on one side of the body or on the face
- rash that's getting bigger or more painful over time
- any new break in the skin that does not heal within a few days (see page 92 for more on leg wounds or page 106 for more on pressure ulcers)

Tips on Providing Relief at Home

If the person develops a rash without warning signs of serious illness:

- Try to identify the cause. Make note of where the rash is on the body, and think about what the person came into contact with or ate recently. Stop using any items or products that you think may be the culprit, and watch to see if the rash gets better.

If the rash is itchy (see below for different tips if the itchy rash is caused by yeast):

- When possible, avoid heat or sunlight and keep the area open to air.
- Try applying a cool, damp washcloth, or bathing the area in cool water, then applying a moisturizer like Vaseline.
- Try an over-the-counter anti-itch cream with hydrocortisone.
- To prevent skin breaks and infection from scratching, keep the person's nails short and the itchy area covered. Try distracting the person with something to hold or listen to. Try having the person wear gloves, especially at night.
- See a health care provider if the rash isn't better in a few days, or if the itching is still severe after trying these tips.

If the person has a skin yeast infection:

- Clean and dry the area at least twice a day. Leave it open to the air if possible.
- After the skin has dried, apply an over-the-counter anti-fungal cream with ketoconazole or clotrimazole.
- If the rash is in the private area and the person is incontinent, encourage healing with frequent diaper changes and an over-the-counter skin protectant like Vaseline, A&D ointment or Desitin.
- See a health care provider if the rash isn't better in a few days.

If the person has stasis dermatitis (rash on lower legs with chronic swelling):

- Clean legs with a mild soap and apply moisturizer every day.
- See page 94 for more on how to improve leg swelling, as this will improve the rash.

Taking Care of Your Own Safety and Stress

Many rashes are not contagious. However, it can be hard to tell if they are. For your safety, use disposable gloves when providing rash care and wash hands often. If the person has shingles, keep the area covered with clothing or a bandage.

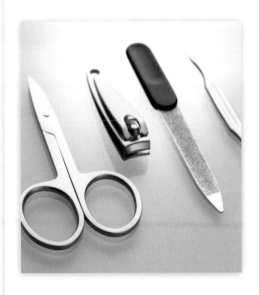

Tip: To prevent skin breaks and infection from scratching, keep the person's nails short and the itchy area covered.

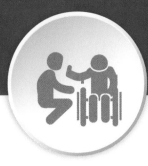

Resisting Personal Care

Basic Facts

Some persons with dementia become upset, uncooperative or even aggressive when being helped with activities like bathing, brushing teeth, or cleaning up after a urine or bowel accident. There are many possible reasons for the behavior, including feeling embarrassed, anxious, rushed, stressed, out of control, or confused. If you're frustrated, think of their lack of cooperation as the only way for the person to tell you that they're overwhelmed.

As with other behavioral symptoms in persons with dementia, the best solutions involve figuring out the causes. Was something done that caused pain, such as moving a stiff joint? Was the person surprised by something they did not understand? Did the person providing care move too fast, overwhelming the person with dementia? Could the person be ill, tired, hungry, or constipated?

Medicine to treat the problem isn't usually as helpful as careful attention to possible causes and then trying different strategies to decrease these triggers.

Signs of a Possible Emergency

Consider calling 911 or taking the person to an emergency department or health care provider office **SOON** if the person has any of these problems:

- **signs of delirium**
  (see page 48 for more on delirium)

- **signs of dehydration**
  (see page 142 for more on dehydration)

- **vital signs very different from usual**, especially temperature over 101° F
  (see page 135 to learn more about vital signs)

Other Important Signs

Consider contacting a health care provider by phone and/or setting up a medical visit **within 1–3 days if you notice:**

- **sudden upset with personal care and signs of sickness** (like fever, cough, or diarrhea)

- **sudden behavior changes**
  (like sleepiness or weakness)

- **new or worsening upset with personal care** that lasts for more than a day

If the person gets angry or aggressive during care:

- Try to stay calm and reassuring.

- Remove or lock away any unsafe items (guns, knives, heavy items).

- Stop whatever you're doing that's upsetting them. You can try again later.

- Try to calm and distract them with another activity.

- If you can't calm them and it's safe to do so, try giving them space. Unless they're in immediate danger, restraining them can make things worse.

- Get help if you need it.

Tips on Providing Relief at Home

Watch a person with sudden upset during personal care carefully for signs of new illness, pain or a physical need. If these aren't the cause, try different strategies until you find what works for your situation.

If the person won't take an important medicine:

- Try to stay calm and reassuring. Use simple sentences to explain why the medicine is important.

- If you take medicine, take your pills at the same time.

- If they continue to refuse to take their medicine, stop and try again later.

- For more information on medications in persons with dementia, see Chapter 7.

If the person seems stressed by personal care:

- Stay calm and reassuring. Try not to show your frustration. If you need to, step away.

- Break tasks into simple steps using clear language. Give choices when possible.

- Go slowly and explain what you'll do before you do it, especially before you touch them.

- Keep a routine for sleep, meals and personal care activities. If needed, try adjusting the schedule (for example, doing more physically demanding activities in the morning).

- Make sure the person is comfortable and that the space around them is calm, quiet and well lit.

- If these tips don't help, stop what you're doing and offer a calm activity. Try again later.

- If the person has pain during certain personal care activities, consider giving a pain reliever like acetaminophen 2 hours before starting care.

- If the person has signs of depression, including seeming sad or tearful most of the time, see page 58.

- If the person seems slow, tired, or unable to help with care activities, see page 54 for more on decreased activity.

- If the person has untrue thoughts (like they think you're trying to hurt them as you provide care), see page 74 for more on delusions.

If the person becomes upset with care:

- Keep careful watch for signs that they're getting sick (like cough), in pain or have a physical need (like hunger).

- Try the tips on this page to problem solve.

- If the person is still not themselves after 24 hours, consider contacting the provider.

Tip: Keep a routine for sleep, meals and activities.
If needed, try adjusting the schedule.

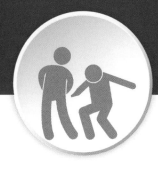

Sexual Behavior Changes

Basic Facts

Changes to the brain with dementia can sometimes mean changes in sexual expression that are new or surprising. For example, the person may show an unusual interest in sex with a spouse or partner; try to touch, hug or kiss strangers; take off clothes in public places; use vulgar language; or even masturbate around others. These behaviors can be very uncomfortable or embarrassing for caregivers.

As with other behavioral symptoms, if the person's sexual behavior changed suddenly, watch for signs of physical illness, pain or a need (like hunger or needing the bathroom). Other times, the behavior is related to being lonely, stressed, confused, or needing physical touch. Whatever the cause, try not to take these behaviors personally. Instead, problem solve to make the best of the situation.

Signs of a Possible Emergency

Consider calling 911 or taking the person to an emergency department or health care provider office **SOON** if the person has any of these problems:

- **you're worried the person may hurt themselves or others**

- **signs of delirium**
  (see page 48 for more on delirium)

- **signs of dehydration**
  (see page 142 for more on dehydration)

- **vital signs very different from usual,** especially temperature over 101° F
  (see page 135 for how to measure vital signs)

Other Important Signs

Consider contacting a health care provider by phone and/or setting up a medical visit **within 1–3 days if you notice:**

- in addition to the new sexual behavior, the person shows signs of physical illness or self-neglect

- the person's sexual behavior is overwhelming to caregivers and/or has a negative effect on their care

- sexual rubbing causes skin problems

If the person has a sudden change in sexual behavior:

- Keep careful watch for signs that they're getting sick (like cough), in pain or have a physical need (like hunger or in need of the bathroom).

- Try the tips on the following page to problem solve.

- If the person is still not themselves after 24 hours, consider contacting the health care provider.

Tips on Providing Relief at Home

A person with sudden changes in sexual behavior should be watched carefully for signs of new illness, pain or a physical need. If these are not the cause, your goal should be to limit behavior that is unsafe, unwanted, or harmful, and accepting any sexual expression that isn't harmful. In all cases, try to stay calm and understanding, rather than scolding the person. If you feel overwhelmed, consider joining a support group and asking a health care provider for help.

If the person takes clothes off or touches private areas around others:

- Check the person for signs of physical need like full bladder, being too hot or cold, or skin rash in the area they're touching.

- Give them something else to do with their hands. Try offering a snack or asking for their help with something.

- If distraction doesn't work, take them to a private area.

- If disrobing happens often, try clothes that fasten in the back.

- Try giving them private time each day to be nude.

If the person touches others in unwanted ways:

- Consistently but calmly tell the person that the behavior isn't appropriate.

- Try to distract the person by giving them something to do with their hands.

- Try offering appropriate physical touch like holding hands, a back rub or hugs.

If the person says inappropriate or vulgar things around others:

- Consistently but calmly tell the person that the behavior isn't appropriate.

- Try changing the topic of conversation or distracting them with an activity.

- Have a pre-prepared card ready that you can give to others explaining the situation, or politely ask others around you to excuse the person's behavior.

- Avoid places that are loud, unfamiliar or stressful.

If the person shows an increased interest in sex:

- Turn down unwanted sexual advances in a firm but respectful way.

- Be cautious about offering appropriate physical touch like holding hands, a back rub or hugs, as it may be misinterpreted.

- Distract the person with an activity they enjoy, or give them space until the mood passes.

- If the person seeks out a new sexual partner in a nursing home or assisted living environment, alert staff and make sure it's consensual. If it's not harmful, it may be best to accept it.

If the person mistakes you for a spouse or sexual partner, gently remind them who you are and see page 74 for more on delusions.

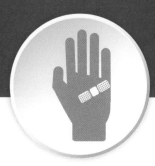

Skin Injuries

Basic Facts

Older people have fragile skin, making skin injuries common even after minor bumps. With careful attention, most skin injuries will heal well at home. There are four main kinds of skin injuries:

- **Cuts:** These happen when something sharp opens the skin. Small cuts can often be cared for at home, while cuts that are deep, wide, on a joint, or that continue to bleed may need medical care.

- **Bruises:** A bruise is bleeding under the skin. They happen more easily when a person is on blood thinning medicines. Most bruises are minor, but a bruise that appears quickly, grows large, or causes severe pain may indicate a serious problem.

- **Scrapes:** These happen when the skin slides across something rough, like a sidewalk. With fragile skin, scrapes can happen when simply sliding across bed sheets.

- **Tears:** A skin tear is a combination of a cut and a scrape and often takes a long time to heal. These happen when the skin twists while a person is being lifted.

If a skin wound is bleeding:

If the person has any urgent warning signs, call 911. While you're waiting for care, or if the bleeding is not too severe:

- Help the person get comfortable.

- Place a clean towel under the area to catch any leaking blood.

- Put firm pressure on the wound for 10 minutes using gauze pads or a clean cloth.

- Check to see if bleeding has stopped. If not, apply pressure for another 15 minutes.

- If the wound continues to bleed after 25 minutes, get medical help.

- If the wound has mostly stopped bleeding, see the next page for how to clean and cover the wound.

Signs of a Possible Emergency

Consider calling 911 or taking the person to an emergency department or health care provider office **SOON** if the person has any of these problems:

- **bleeding that you can't stop** after 15–30 minutes

- **a wide or deep wound** that may need stitches

- a possible **broken bone or a deep wound** that may reach the bone. Signs include:

  - Severe pain, the person can't move the area

  - You see bone

  - Serious injury over a joint

- **head injuries** with urgent signs (see page 76)

- **injuries with dirt, glass or other material that you can't get out**

Other Important Signs

Consider contacting a health care provider by phone and/or setting up a medical visit **within 1–3 days if you notice:**

- signs of skin infection or poor healing (see next page)

- injuries that may be the result of abuse or neglect (see page 28)

Tips on Providing Relief at Home

If the person has a bruise:

- Apply ice (wrapped in a towel) on and off every 20–30 minutes for the first day or so. A bag of frozen peas or other vegetables works well if you don't have an ice pack.

- If possible, have the person rest and raise the area.

If the person has a skin tear or an open wound:

- Stop bleeding by applying pressure with a clean gauze or cloth.

- For open wounds, gently clean the area once a day with warm water or saline and a mild soap. For skin tears, do this every two days.

- For skin tears, try to put the skin 'flap' back in place with gauze.

- Apply a layer of Vaseline or antibiotic ointment.

- Cover the wound with a non-stick bandage like Telfa. Try to avoid putting tape directly on the skin by wrapping the area with dry gauze or an Ace bandage.

- If you have a smartphone, take photos of the area to show or send to the health care provider.

For all skin injury care and prevention:

- For temporary pain relief, use acetaminophen (Tylenol) or another pain medication recommended by the health care provider. Don't give aspirin, BC, or Goody powders as these can make bleeding worse.

- Make sure the person is up-to-date on their tetanus shot (within 10 years).

- To protect the skin from bumps and scrapes:

  - Have the person wear long sleeves/pants and high thick socks.

  - Use skin moisturizer twice a day.

  - Pad furniture edges.

  - Keep your nails short and avoid wearing sharp jewelry while providing daily care.

- A healthy diet full of fruit, vegetables, and proteins will help the skin stay strong and heal.

What to Watch Out For

- **Skin Infection:** In the days to weeks after a skin injury, contact the health care provider if you notice any of these changes:

  - Fever

  - New or increasing wound:

    - Swelling

    - Redness

    - Pain or tenderness

    - Warmth

    - Drainage (fluid or pus coming out)

- **Poor healing:** Contact the health care provider if:

  - a wound is not any better after 1 week

  - there is new or continuing bleeding

  - a bruise continues to grow even with icing and resting the area

Taking Care of Your Own Safety and Stress

- Wash your hands thoroughly before and after cleaning a wound or changing bandages. If possible, wear disposable gloves when providing care.

See Chapter 3 for more ways to take care of yourself.

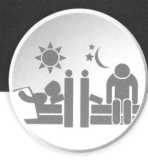

Sleep Problems—Daytime

Basic Facts

Many persons with dementia suffer from one or more problems with daytime sleep, such as falling asleep during daily activities; needing naps to get through the day; or feeling sluggish, irritable or agitated from being overtired. If there's a sudden change in daytime sleep, it could be a sign of a new or worsening illness (like a virus). Other more gradual causes of daytime sleep problems include:

- Poor sleep at night (see page 118 for more on nighttime sleep problems)
- Not being physically active
- Not getting enough bright light (often due to not going outside)
- Not having routine sleep and wake times
- Dementia-related problems with the body's "internal clock," which can be worsened by low physical activity or low light exposure during the day, or by not having a routine bedtime
- Side effects of medications

Although most daytime sleep problems are not emergencies, they can impact the person's mood, well-being, and how well they sleep at night. Treating these problems can bring relief for both the person with dementia and those they live with.

Signs of a Possible Emergency

Consider calling 911 or taking the person to an emergency department or health care provider office **SOON** if the person has any of these problems:

- **you can't wake the person up**
- **increased sleepiness with trouble breathing**
- **signs of delirium** (see page 48 for more on delirium)
- **vital signs very different from usual**, especially temperature above 101° F (see page 135 for how to measure vital signs)

Other Important Signs

Consider contacting a health care provider by phone and/or setting up a medical visit **within 1–3 days if:**

- you notice increased daytime sleep with signs of a new or worsening illness
- the person with dementia is still driving and you're worried they might fall asleep at the wheel
- sleep problems are causing stress in the home
- the person has signs of "sundowning" (see page 49)
- the person **often stops breathing while sleeping** (see page 118 for more on sleep apnea)

If the person seems unusually sleepy or difficult to awaken:

- Watch them for signs of a new or worsening illness.
- Try to wake them by gently rubbing their arm or back, or by putting lights on or opening the blinds.
- Once awake, measure the person's vital signs. If they are abnormal, consider contacting a health care provider.
- See "tips" on the next page for ways to encourage healthy sleep.

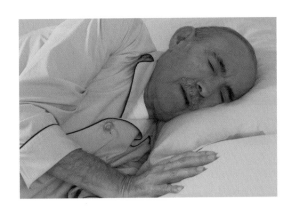

Tips on Providing Relief at Home

Every person's sleep needs are different, and some need more sleep than others. The "right" amount of sleep allows the person to feel rested and be a part of enjoyable daily activities.

Tips to encourage healthy sleep patterns:

- If daytime sleepiness is a new problem, look for a cause such as a medicine side effect, a new illness, or a change in their routine.

- If the person is also having trouble with nighttime sleep, see page 118.

- Bring the person outside or by windows where they can be around natural light at least 15 minutes a day. Bright light is especially helpful in the morning.

- Help regulate the body's internal clock by keeping a daily routine with regular wake, meal and bed times.

- Offer activities they enjoy and physical movement throughout the day.

- Avoid alcohol and smoking. Limit caffeine and sweets to early in the day. Offer a larger lunch and a light dinner.

- Try encouraging a short (30 minute) nap in the afternoon. If it's helpful, try to stick to a routine naptime each day.

- At night, dim lights (keeping some lights on for safety) and encourage quiet, relaxing activities before bedtime.

- Help the person stay up until their usual bedtime.

What to Watch Out For

- **Delirium:** Delirium is a sudden worsening of confusion that can be a sign of a serious illness. The person may quickly (over hours) change back and forth between alert, hyperactive and sleepy.

  - See page 48 for more on delirium.

  - Consider getting medical help right away.

- **"Sundowning":** This refers to a common condition in persons with dementia – becoming more agitated or confused toward the end of the day. Common causes include exhaustion, decreased sunlight, and increased activity around the house.

  - Keep the home well lit.

  - Encourage quiet evening activities.

  - See page 30 for more on agitation.

- **Mood changes:** If the person has sleep problems and also seems sad, worried, angry, or doesn't want to do things they once enjoyed, they may be suffering from depression (page 58).

  - Keep unsafe objects (like knives) locked or out of the home.

Taking Care of Your Own Safety and Stress

If the person's sleep problems are making it hard for you to get restful sleep, ask a health care provider for help.

See Chapter 3 for more ways to take care of yourself.

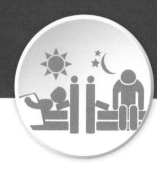

Sleep Problems—Nighttime

Basic Facts

A person with nighttime sleep problems may have trouble falling or staying asleep, or they may be waking up very early or late. Sometimes, these problems are due to a dementia-related upset to the body's "internal clock," making day and night mixed up. These problems are made worse by not getting much physical activity or natural light and by sleeping during the day.

Another cause of poor sleep at night can be a medical sleep problem, such as:

- **Sleep apnea:** If the person snores loudly and seems to stop breathing or gasp for air while asleep, they may not be getting enough oxygen to the brain. This can make the person feel tired or irritable during the day, and can lead to heart disease and other problems. If you're concerned, talk to a provider who can test for and treat this problem.

- **Restless legs:** In this treatable condition, the person has nighttime leg twitching or jerking.

- **Nighttime wandering:** Sometimes wandering at night is part of the upset "internal clock," but it could also be a sign of things like pain, heart problems, or needing to use the bathroom.

- **Sleepwalking or night terrors:** In this case, the person is acting out dreams or doing odd things while asleep. In night terrors, the person may be very upset or even violent. This is especially common in persons with Lewy body dementia.

Signs of a Possible Emergency

Consider calling 911 or taking the person to an emergency department or health care provider office **SOON** if the person has any of these problems:

- you can't wake the person up

- increased sleepiness with fever or trouble breathing

- signs of delirium (see page 48 for more on delirium)

- vital signs very different from usual (see page 135 for how to measure vital signs)

Other Important Signs

Consider contacting a health care provider by phone and/or setting up a medical visit **within 1–3 days if you notice:**

- changes in nighttime sleep with any signs of a new or worsening illness

- the person **often stops breathing while sleeping**

- **night terrors or nightmares** where the person is very upset and hard to comfort

If the person has night terrors:

- Keep unsafe items locked or out of the home.
- Stay calm and close by.
- Try comforting them with gentle touch or calming music.
- Check for signs that the person is uncomfortable (needing to use the bathroom, too hot or cold, in pain).
- Tell the provider about the episode, especially if it happens often.

Tips on Providing Relief at Home

Here are some tips to encourage healthy sleep patterns:

- If nighttime sleep problems are new, consider whether medicine side effects, a new illness, or a change in their routine could be the cause.

- Daytime sleep habits (page 116) can have a big impact on nighttime sleep.

  - Avoid alcohol and smoking. Limit caffeine and sweets to early in the day.

  - Encourage outside time or sitting near a window for natural light every day.

  - Have routine wake, afternoon nap (if helpful) and sleep times. Avoid going to bed before it's time.

  - Encourage regular body movement and enjoyable activities throughout the day.

  - At night, dim the lights and encourage a quiet, relaxing nighttime routine.

  - Unless you're concerned about dehydration, offer less fluid in the 2–3 hours before bed.

  - Keep the sleeping area comfortable (quiet, dark or dim, good temperature).

If the person wanders or sleepwalks at night:

- Keep bedrooms, hallways and stairs lit, or have motion sensors that turn on lights with movement.

- Keep all walk areas clear of things that could be tripped on (including throw rugs).

- Put bells, chimes, or an alarm on doors to unsafe areas. Dead bolting a door should be a last resort.

- If you sleep in a different room, consider using a baby monitor to keep track of when the person gets up.

- Put labels and signs around the house to help the person find things such as the bathroom.

- Keep dangerous items (knives, guns, cleaning supplies) locked or out of the home.

- Lock or take knobs off of the stove.

What to Watch Out For

- **Side effects from sleep medicines:** Persons with dementia can have many problems from sleep medicines including:

  - More falls

  - More confusion

  - More daytime sleepiness

Ask a health care provider for advice before using any sleep aids.

Taking Care of Your Own Safety and Stress

If the person's sleep problems are making it hard for you to get restful nighttime sleep:

- As best as you can, keep your own regular wake and sleep schedules.

- Allow yourself to nap during the day. Keep daytime naps brief (30 minutes or less).

- Ask a family member, friend, or neighbor to fill in for you 1 or 2 nights per week so that you can get the sleep you need.

- Talk to the health care provider for advice.

See Chapter 3 for more ways to take care of yourself.

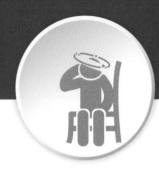

Stroke

Basic Facts

A stroke happens when the brain is damaged due to a blocked artery ("ischemic stroke") or bleeding ("hemorrhagic stroke"). Stroke is often treatable if caught early; so knowing the stroke signs and getting medical treatment as soon as possible can save brain cells. Dementia can be caused by or made worse by one or more strokes.

Older persons can also have "transient ischemic attacks" (TIAs), also known as "mini-strokes," where blood flow is interrupted for a short time. In this case, the person may have warning signs that come suddenly and then go away within a few minutes or hours. However, even if signs of stroke go away, it's important to get medical help right away. "Mini-strokes" can lead to a full blown stroke if not treated.

Signs of a Possible Emergency

Consider calling 911 or taking the person to an emergency department or health care provider office **SOON** if the person has any of these problems:

- **sudden numbness or weakness of the face (drooping), arm, or leg,** especially if on one side of the body

- **sudden confusion, trouble speaking or understanding speech**

- **sudden trouble seeing** in one or both eyes

- **sudden trouble walking, dizziness, loss of balance, coordination, or unexplained falls**

- **sudden severe headache**

- **any signs above that come and go** (even if lasting only a few minutes)

If you're concerned the person may be having a stroke:

- Ask the person to smile.
  Does one side of their face droop?

- Ask the person a question.
  Does their speech sound suddenly slurred?

- Ask the person to raise their arms.
  Does one side lift higher than the other?

If you answered "Yes" to any of these questions, a stroke may be happening. Consider **calling 911** right away.

Tips on Providing Relief at Home

After a stroke, the person may have lasting problems in different parts of the body, depending on the area of the brain affected.

If the person has trouble speaking, communicating or understanding speech:

- The person may find this frustrating. Try to be patient and ignore mistakes.

- Speak slowly and directly, giving them plenty of time to respond.

- If the person has trouble answering questions, try only asking "yes" or "no" questions.

  - See page 128 for more on voice and speaking problems.

If the person has trouble swallowing or eating:

- Have them sit upright to eat.

- Avoid distractions, such as talking, during meals.

- Try offering softer foods or purees and encourage them to swallow before taking another bite.

- See page 46 for more on chewing and swallowing and page 98 for more on not eating or drinking.

If the person is having trouble moving around:

- Prevent accidents by doing a safety check of the home. This includes removing tripping hazards, adding grab bars where needed, and keeping living areas well-lit.

- See page 68 for more on preventing falls.

To decrease the chances of another stroke, encourage the person to:

- quit smoking

- eat a healthy diet low in saturated fat,

- stay as physically active as possible, and

- take medicines if needed to control high blood pressure, high cholesterol or diabetes.

What to Watch Out For

- **Another stroke:** People who have had a stroke are at risk for another. Get medical help right away if they have any sudden new or worsening stroke warning signs.

- **Easy bleeding or bruising:** After a stroke, the person may be placed on a blood thinning medicine that can make bleeding more likely. Talk to the health care provider if you notice:

  - Unexplained bruising

  - Bleeding from gums or nose

  - Blood in urine

  - Black, tarry, or cranberry colored stool

  - A fall (they are more likely to have bleeding with injuries)

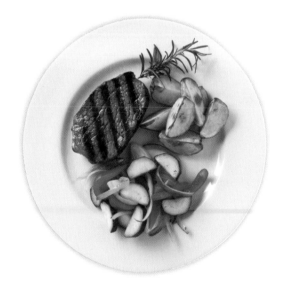

Tip: Eat a healthy diet low in saturated fat.

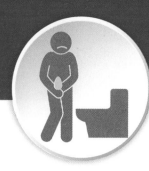

Urine Accidents (Incontinence)

Basic Facts

Urine accidents (or incontinence) are common in dementia, especially as the disease progresses. Some causes are treatable, like medication side effects, urinary infections, or constipation. However, dementia often causes a slow, progressive loss of bladder control that begins with frequent, sudden urges to go. This problem is made worse by things like trouble getting to the bathroom. Weakness of the muscles around the bladder and trouble emptying the bladder completely are two other common problems that can lead to accidents. Eventually, dementia takes away all bladder control, to a point that sometimes people with advanced dementia don't even realize when they are urinating.

Luckily, urine incontinence is not usually an urgent problem, but it's important to report new or worsening incontinence to a health care provider, as many causes can be treated or made better.

Signs of a Possible Emergency

Consider calling 911 or taking the person to an emergency department or health care provider office **SOON** if the person has any of these problems:

- **shaking chills**

- **severe lower belly or lower back pain** (the person is doubled over, crying, or can't move)

- the person **can't urinate** (except for small amounts), despite feeling like they have to

- the person **pulled out a bladder catheter**

- **signs of delirium** (see page 48 for more on delirium)

- **vital signs very different from usual**, especially temperature above 101° F (see page 135 for how to measure vital signs)

Other Important Signs

Consider contacting a health care provider by phone and/or setting up a medical visit **within 1–3 days if a person with new or worsening urine incontinence ALSO has:**

- **temperature above 99° F** or 1.2° F above the person's normal body temperature (see page 70 for more on fever) and/or **lower belly or lower back pain** or **painful urination**

- **blood in the urine**

- **red, raw or open skin** on the thighs or private areas in a person with urine or bowel accidents

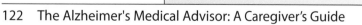

Tips on Providing Relief at Home

Urine accidents are a part of dementia and not something the person can control.

Here are some tips to make accidents less stressful:

- Keep offering at least 6 cups of fluid every day. Holding back fluid can cause the person to become dehydrated and increase the risk for falls, infections, and worsening confusion. However, if the person has accidents at night, it's okay to avoid drinks for three hours before bedtime.

- Try to stay calm and compassionate as you help.

- Provide clothing with Velcro straps or elastic waistbands; they'll be easy to pull down or remove.

- Install a raised toilet seat to make it easier to get on and off the toilet.

- Encourage the person to be as independent as they can. Give step-by-step directions and reassurance when needed.

  - If you are helping in the bathroom, give the person plenty of time. If the person seems uncomfortable with you being there, step out or look the other way.

  - If the person needs your help but is uncooperative, see the section on resisting personal care (page 110).

If the person has some control but sometimes has "accidents":

- Make sure the path to the bathroom is clear of barriers and is well lit at all times. Keep the bathroom door open to make getting there easier.

- Watch for signs that the person needs to go to the bathroom and remind them to go, or else remind them to go on a schedule, such as every two hours.

- Keep a record of when they urinate so you get to know their habits.

- Give praise and encouragement when the person stays dry or uses the toilet.

- If the person is unstable on their feet, provide a walking aid and/or grab bars.

- If the person has trouble getting to the bathroom, use a bedside commode, urinal, or bed pan.

If the person is incontinent frequently:

- Wash and dry the skin after each accident; adult wipes make clean-up easier. After cleaning, prevent skin problems by applying an over-the-counter cream such as Vaseline, A&D Ointment, or Desitin.

- Have the person use absorbent pads or briefs. It will take some trial and error to figure out which works best.

- Use disposable pads to protect the bedding and prevent unnecessary linen changes. Rubberized flannel baby sheets can also be used.

Taking Care of Your Own Safety and Stress

To protect you and the person you are providing care for:

- Wear disposable gloves when helping the person use the bathroom or cleaning up accidents.

- Wash your hands before and after helping the person with bathroom needs.

- Use appropriate lifting techniques if helping the person stand or sit up in bed (see page 16).

See Chapter 3 for more ways to take care of yourself.

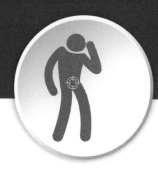

Basic Facts

It is often normal for some bacteria to live in an older person's bladder. In fact, over 50% of older persons have bacteria in their bladders without any symptoms or problems. However, certain germs can lead to urinary tract infection (UTI) in the bladder or kidney. When this happens, the person may have pain or burning with urination, pain in the lower belly or back, blood in the urine, fever, or they may urinate more often or have more urine accidents.

Sometimes, you or the health care provider may suspect a UTI because the person is acting differently—perhaps they're not eating well or they just don't seem themselves. In the past, antibiotics were given "just in case" of UTI. But now we know that most of the time such "nonspecific" symptoms are caused by other things, such as pain, anxiety, constipation, poor sleep, or dehydration. Also, we worry more about the side effects from giving antibiotics too often. For these reasons, if the person is not having clear UTI symptoms, most health care providers now look for other problems and/or wait to see if the person gets better on their own before giving an antibiotic.

Signs of a Possible Emergency

Consider calling 911 or taking the person to an emergency department or health care provider office **SOON** if the person has any of these problems:

- **shaking chills**
- **severe lower belly or lower back pain** (the person is doubled over, crying, or can't move)
- **blood clots** in the urine
- the person **can't urinate** (except for small amounts), despite feeling like they have to
- **signs of delirium** (see page 48 for more on delirium)
- **vital signs very different from usual,** especially temperature above 101° F (see page 135 for how to measure vital signs)

Other Important Signs

Consider contacting a health care provider by phone and/or setting up a medical visit **within 1–3 days if you notice:**

- **symptoms lasting longer than 7 days**
- **temperature above 99° F** or 1.2° F above the person's normal body temperature (see page 70 for more on fever) and/or **lower belly or lower back pain** or **painful urination**
- **blood in the urine**
- **pus or fluid** from the vagina or penis
- **sudden changes in urinary habits** (new or increasing urine accidents, going to the bathroom more often) without any other cause, lasting for more than 4 days

Tips on Providing Relief at Home

Here are some things you can do at home if the person has a UTI. In all cases, offer at least 6 cups of fluid every day to help prevent dehydration. The urine should be clear or light yellow in color.

If the person is having pain with urination, lower belly or lower back pain:

- Offer acetaminophen (Tylenol) or other pain reliever recommended by a health care provider.
- Apply a heating pad to the painful area.

If the person is having trouble "going"/urinating (urine retention):

- Make sure they are drinking enough fluids to produce urine.
- Give privacy and plenty of time in the bathroom.
- Turn on the faucet, place the person's hands in warm water, or run warm water over the private area while they try to urinate.
- Encourage them to lean forward and/or gently push on their belly while on the toilet.
- Get medical help right away if they've gotten little or no urine out after 8 hours, especially if they also have worsening lower belly pain.

If the person is having urine accidents or sudden urges to urinate (see page 122):

- Every two hours or so, ask the person if they need to use the bathroom.
- Keep the bathroom door open and light on. Have the person wear simple clothing (with an elastic waist). If needed, try a bedside commode or bedpan.
- Dry the person after an accident. Wetness can be uncomfortable and causes skin problems.
- Continue to offer at least 6 cups of fluid each day. If they have nighttime accidents, don't offer drinks in the 3 hours before bedtime.
- If they can't tell you they need to urinate, look for clues. They may say certain things, start to pace, or get suddenly worried when they need to go.

Collecting a "Clean" Urine Sample Using a "Collection Hat"

If the person cannot easily provide a clean sample, obtain a "collection hat" from a health care provider or drug store. After drinking fluid, have the person sit on the toilet and clean the genital area as well as you can. In women, wipe with an antiseptic towellete from front to back, spreading the vaginal folds. In men, wipe the tip of the penis while holding back any foreskin. Have the person urinate as usual (avoid any stool). Afterwards, wearing gloves, pour the urine from the hat into a collection cup. Tell the provider that the sample was collected in a hat.

If the person has a bladder catheter:

- Make sure there aren't kinks in the tubing and that urine is going into the bag.
- If the person is pulling at the catheter, keep the catheter out of sight by covering it with clothing. Offer a distraction.

If you're trying to prevent UTIs:

- Offer at least 6 cups of fluids each day.
- When wiping the vagina, move front to back, so you don't get bowel bacteria in the vagina.
- Try cranberry juice or tablets, which have been shown to prevent some infections. Check that the person isn't taking any medications that shouldn't be taken with cranberry juice.
- Encourage the person to use the bathroom regularly (about every two hours).
- Wash and dry the skin after each accident.

Taking Care of Your Own Safety and Stress

For your protection, wear disposable gloves when helping with personal care.

See Chapter 3 for more ways to take care of yourself.

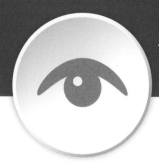

Vision Problems

Basic Facts

When a person with dementia can't see well, it can keep them from doing things they enjoy and increase confusion. Small improvements in vision can make a big difference. For these reasons, it's worth having vision checked regularly or if you notice signs of trouble seeing.

Most vision problems in older people happen slowly. They can be due to normal changes in the eyes with age or diseases such as cataracts, glaucoma, macular degeneration, or diabetes. In addition, dementia can damage the brain's ability to recognize things (like faces or colors), notice movement, judge depth, or understand where the body is. In daily life, the person with vision trouble may bump into things, mistake one thing for another, or have trouble reaching for things.

Meanwhile, sudden vision loss is an emergency, as it can mean a problem with eye blood flow, pressure inside the eye, or the nerve at the back of the eye. The person may or may not have other symptoms like eye redness or pain, headache or nausea. In any case, getting help right away can save eyesight.

Signs of a Possible Emergency

Consider calling 911 or taking the person to an emergency department or health care provider office **SOON** if the person has any of these problems:

- **sudden vision loss**

- **sudden loss or change in vision** (blurry vision, double vision, light flashes, new "floaters") **in one or both eyes**, with or without **eye pain, eye redness, nausea or vomiting**

- **headaches on both temples** that don't go away with pain medication, especially if the person is also having vision changes

- **light suddenly bothers the eye(s) a lot** (the person may need to wear sunglasses inside)

Other Important Signs

Consider contacting an eye care provider by phone and/or setting up a medical visit **within 1–3 days if you notice new trouble with:**

- recognizing faces or reading facial expressions

- seeing in low or bright light, or both

- finding things

- reading or enjoying familiar hobbies

- managing in unfamiliar or familiar areas

- finding food on the plate

- managing current glasses, or saying "I need new glasses."

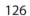

Tips on Providing Relief at Home

Here are some tips for making daily life easier for the person with vision trouble:

- Make everyday objects bigger by using things like large print books or by moving their chair closer to the television.

- Have bright lighting available, like a reading lamp, for looking at things up close. You might try a hand magnifier with an LED light.

- Use different colored objects to make them stand out. For example, at mealtime put white pasta on a dark plate. Then, use a white placemat to make the edges of the dark plate stand out.

- Remove mirrors or shiny surfaces if they cause confusion.

- Close the curtains or blinds to prevent glare.

- Keep the living space safe by:

  - Offering your arm for guidance as the person walks.

  - Providing bright, even lighting especially in areas like hallways, stairways and bathrooms.

  - Marking the edges of things like stairs, furniture or doorways with brightly colored tape.

  - Removing tripping hazards from walkways and avoiding busy floor or wall patterns.

- Have the person's vision checked regularly.

- Encourage the person to wear their glasses, and check that they're clean and that the prescription is correct. For most persons with dementia, having separate glasses for distance and reading is safer than bifocals.

- If the person is upset by their vision trouble:

  - Try not to bring attention to mistakes or to argue with them if they see something incorrectly.

  - When possible, modify activities so they can still enjoy them (like using audio books).

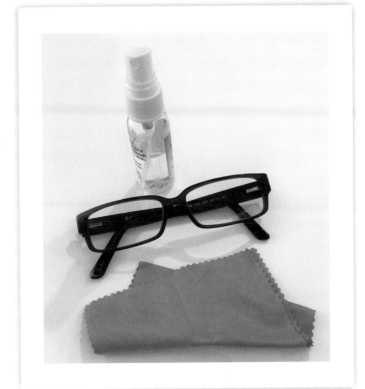

What to Watch Out For

- **Falls:** Difficulty seeing can make falls more likely. The person may move slowly because of fear of falling.

  - Use the tips on this page for making the living space safe.

  - See page 68 for more on falls.

- **Not eating or drinking:** If the person can't see well, they may not eat or drink even when the food is placed in front of them.

  - Use color to make food and drink stand out.

  - Help the person recognize food and utensils, and help them to use them if needed.

  - See page 98 for more on not eating or drinking, and for signs of dehydration.

Voice and Speaking Problems

Basic Facts

A person with a new voice problem may have a voice that's weak, hoarse, or scratchy. Often, the problem is from irritation of the vocal cords from a virus (called laryngitis), allergy, smoking, talking too much, or acid reflux. Changes to the voice can also be caused by medications, or weakening of throat muscles in dementia and other brain conditions. More rarely, changes to the voice can be a sign of throat cancer.

If the speaking problem is caused by a brain disease, the person may also have trouble understanding language, word finding, or making their mouth move. If these problems happen suddenly, they can be a sign of stroke.

Signs of a Possible Emergency

Consider calling 911 or taking the person to an emergency department or health care provider office **SOON** if the person has any of these problems:

- signs of a **stroke**, including: (see page 120 for more on stroke)
  - **sudden trouble speaking (slurring, mumbling, can't find words), reading, writing, or understanding others**
  - **face droops or looks uneven**
  - **new weakness or numbness in a body part**
- **coughing up a large amount of blood** (more than 1 cup in 24 hours)
- **severe shortness of breath** or **trouble breathing** (see page 40 for more on breathing problems)
- **new severe trouble swallowing** (the person may drool or lean forward to breathe)
- **severe headache or stiff neck**
- **seizures or passing out** (see page 104 for more on passing out)
- **voice or speaking problems** after an injury or surgery
- **signs of delirium** (see page 48 for more on delirium)
- **vital signs very different from usual** (see page 135 for how to measure vital signs)

Other Important Signs

Consider contacting a health care provider by phone and/or setting up a medical visit **within 1–3 days if a person has a voice problem AND has:**

- **sudden voice loss or voice changes lasting 2 or more weeks**
- **painful speaking or swallowing**
- **sore throat with fever**
- the person is **sad, worried or agitated** because of the voice or speaking problems
- **unintentional weight loss**

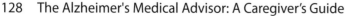

Tips on Providing Relief at Home

If the person has voice problems:

- Gently encourage the person to rest their voice. Offer activities that don't require talking, like watching a show or listening to music.

- Use a humidifier or a steam vaporizer, or encourage the person to take a steamy shower (if this doesn't upset them).

- Offer at least 6 cups of fluids they enjoy each day.

- Avoid things that can make voice problems worse like smoke, dust, pollen and pets. If they can't be avoided, try using a face mask (if this doesn't upset them).

- If the voice problems are due to heartburn:

  - Limit high fat foods, chocolate, coffee, colas, acidic juices (like orange juice), and alcohol.

  - Don't eat or drink for 3 hours before lying down.

  - Raise the head of the bed 6–8 inches.

If you have trouble communicating with someone due to speaking problems:

- Keep distractions and noise to a minimum.

- Use simple sentences and give the person time to respond.

- If you don't understand what the person is trying to say, ask them to clarify with a yes/no question ("Did you say you'd like water?").

- Try different ways to communicate, like writing, drawing, and gesturing. If the person is in early stages of dementia, try a non-verbal communication board (available at medical supply stores).

- Encourage the person to speak, even if it takes a lot of time. Try to be patient and ignore mistakes. Let the person know that you understand their frustration.

What to Watch Out For

- **Mood or behavior changes:** Not being able to communicate well can cause the person to feel sad, worried or angry. See the guides on agitation (page 30), anger (page 32), anxiety (page 34) and/or depression (page 58) for more information.

- **Swallowing problems:** A person with voice or speaking problems may also have swallowing difficulty. This makes choking and lung infections more likely. See page 46 for more on swallowing.

Taking Care of Your Own Safety and Stress

- If the person has an infection, wash your hands often. If the person is coughing, ask them to wear a mask. If they can't or won't wear one, wear one yourself.

- If the person is aggressive due to problems communicating, remove or lock away unsafe items. If needed, get help.

See Chapter 3 for more ways to take care of yourself.

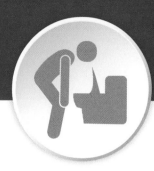

Vomiting

Basic Facts

Vomiting, or throwing up, is most often caused by an infection with a virus or bacteria ("stomach bug"), food poisoning, or from a reaction to a medicine like antibiotics or pain relievers. Sometimes, vomiting occurs just because a food or drink did not agree with the person, and afterward they are fine. Other times, vomiting can be caused by a more serious problem in the belly (like gallstones or a blockage in the intestines), in the chest (like a heart attack on pneumonia), or in the brain (like a stroke). Also, sometimes a person throws up when they have severe pain or are worried.

It's important to keep close watch on someone who's vomiting. Although many causes of vomiting can be cared for at home, if the person has warning signs of a serious problem, get medical help.

Signs of a Possible Emergency

Consider calling 911 or taking the person to an emergency department or health care provider office **SOON** if the person has any of these problems:

- severe belly pain, or pain that gets worse over time
- belly is **swollen**, **hard** or **very tender** to the touch
- vomit that looks bloody or like "coffee grounds"
- vomiting that is preceded by severe headache, chest pain, or difficulty breathing
- seizure
- signs of dehydration (see page 142 for more on dehydration)
- signs of delirium (see page 48 for more on delirium)
- vital signs very different from usual, especially temperature above 101° F (see page 135 for how to measure vital signs)

Other Important Signs

Consider contacting a health care provider by phone and/or setting up a medical visit **within 1–3 days if a person has been vomiting AND you notice:**

- low-grade fever for longer than 48 hours (see page 70 for more on fever)
- vomiting lasting more than 24 hours
- diarrhea lasting more than 2 days (even if vomiting has stopped)
- yellow skin or yellow whites of eyes (even if vomiting has stopped)
- not eating or drinking well (even if vomiting has stopped)
- any other thing that makes you worried that the person isn't right

Tips on Providing Relief at Home

Here are some things you can do at home for vomiting:

- Slowly offer fluids. Aim for 6 or more cups each day (avoid alcohol and drinks high in caffeine).

  - Try sports drinks, like Gatorade. These help put salt and sugar back in the body. Water and juices are also okay.

  - Offer small sips every few minutes instead of big gulps.

  - If the person throws up after drinking even small amounts, try giving just 1–3 tablespoons of fluid every 15 minutes.

- Wait at least 6–12 hours after vomiting before offering light solid food. Some good options include crackers, toast, and rice. If solid foods make the vomiting worse, stick with fluids until the vomiting stops.

- To help prevent choking, encourage the person to lean over or lie on their side when vomiting. Keep a bucket nearby.

- After the person has thrown up, help them feel comfortable and clean. Offer a tissue for blowing the nose. Offer a small amount of water as a mouth rinse. Help them to brush their teeth.

- If the vomiting is stressful or frequent, try an anti-vomiting medicine. Pepto-Bismol is an over-the-counter remedy that can help. Keep in mind, however, that if the person has stomach flu, vomiting is the body's way of getting rid of the virus.

- If you've tried these tips and the person is still vomiting after 12 hours, see the health care provider.

What to Watch Out For

- **Low fluid in the body (dehydration):** A person with dementia can quickly become dehydrated. Signs of dehydration are:

  - Dry mouth and tongue

  - Urinating very little

  - Fast heart beat

  - Slow, weak, or low energy

If you've tried the tips on this page but the person still seems dehydrated or isn't keeping fluids down, get medical help.

- **Lung infection (pneumonia):** Vomit can get into the lungs and cause pneumonia. Bring the person to the health care provider if you notice:

  - Breathing faster than usual

  - New noisy breathing

  - Coughing

  - Fever

- **Teeth problems:** Vomit has acids that can hurt the teeth. Be sure to:

  - Have the person rinse their mouth out after vomiting

  - Brush and floss the teeth often

Taking Care of Your Own Safety and Stress

- Wash your hands often and wear gloves when cleaning up vomit. Use germ-killing cleansers.

See Chapter 3 for more ways to take care of yourself.

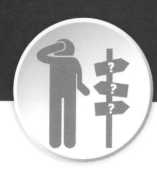

Wandering

Basic Facts

When a person with dementia wanders, it can be stressful for others. The person may pace, try to open locked doors, follow someone around the home, or get lost in the neighborhood or beyond. The person may wander because they're confused, looking for something, worried, convinced they need to be somewhere, or just bored.

As with other behavioral symptoms, medicines to treat wandering don't usually help. The best strategies for dealing with wandering include making the inside of the home safe, preventing the person from wandering outside of the home, and being prepared in case the person does wander outside and gets lost.

Signs of a Possible Emergency

Consider calling 911 or taking the person to an emergency department or health care provider office **SOON** if the person has any of these problems:

- **the person has wandered off, you've found them in a dangerous place, and you can't convince them to return**

- signs of delirium
  (see page 48 for more on delirium)

- signs of dehydration
  (see page 142 for more on dehydration)

- vital signs very different from usual, especially temperature over 101° F
  (see page 135 for how to measure vital signs)

Other Important Signs

Consider contacting a health care provider by phone and/or setting up a medical visit **within 1–3 days if you notice:**

- **wandering with signs that the person may be getting sick** (like fever, cough, or diarrhea)

- **new or worsening wandering** lasting more than a day

If the person is lost:

- Take 15–20 minutes to search carefully where the person was last seen.

- Get help searching from family, friends, neighbors or anyone nearby right away.

- If you don't find the person in 15–20 minutes, call 911 and keep searching.

- When you find the person, comfort them and try not to show anger.

- If you called the police, let them know that the person has been found.

- Check the person for injuries. Get medical help if needed.

- When the person is safe, think about the possible causes of the wandering and make a prevention plan.

Tips on Providing Relief at Home

Wandering can be dangerous and even life-threatening. Use these tips to help keep the person safe.

If the person insists on leaving the house:

- Try figuring out why they want to leave. For example, if they're looking for something, perhaps you can help them find it.

- Try distracting them with a snack, by asking them to help you with something, or by offering an activity they enjoy.

- Give the person a reason to stay. You might say something like: "It's cold out. Let's read instead."

- If you can't persuade them to stay, don't argue, as this will likely make them more upset.

- If possible, join them outside for a walk. After a while, you can circle back home.

- If the person insists on leaving and it's not safe to walk, get help from someone else.

Make sure the home is safe for wandering:

- Keep dangerous things such as guns, knives, glass, and sharp or heavy objects, and chemicals like cleaning supplies, out of the house or locked away.

- Make sure that stairs have good lighting and railings.

- Make the stove safe by removing the knobs or putting a lock on the gas or electricity.

- Use a baby monitor to keep track of the person.

- Use nightlights to make night wandering safer.

- Install bells, chimes or alarms on doors that open to the outside.

Be prepared in case of a wandering emergency:

- Keep something on the person that shows who they are and your phone number. This could be an ID card, a bracelet or labels on clothing. A good option is the Alzheimer's Association Safe Return Program.

- Always carry a current photo of the person and their key medical information to give to the police.

- Keep a list of phone numbers of people who can help you right away if the person goes missing.

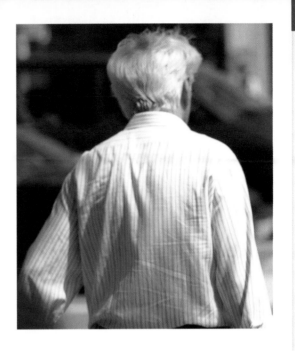

What to Watch Out For

- **Falls:** Wandering puts the person at risk for a fall. See page 68 for more on how to prevent falls and what to do if the person has fallen.

- **Aggression:** Sometimes keeping a person from leaving the home can lead to aggression. See page 32 for more on managing aggression.

'' The doctor wanted me to check
dad's blood pressure a few times a
week, but dad wouldn't sit still.
I figured out that if I did it when he
was watching TV, I'd have the job
done before he knew it.

— *Christine L., caregiver*

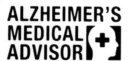

**ALZHEIMER'S
MEDICAL [+]
ADVISOR**

Keeping an Eye on Medical Issues and General Health

Measuring and Understanding Vital Signs

Vital signs are measurements of the body's most basic functions; they include **pulse, breathing rate, body temperature** and **blood pressure**. With some training and a few tools, they can easily be measured at home.

Measuring and recording vital signs routinely allows you to know the person's "normal" or typical vital sign range. By comparing usual measurements to measurements taken when the person may be sick or injured, you'll be gathering important information about the severity of the problem. Vital signs can help you and the health care provider decide between home monitoring, an office visit, or urgent care. See Chapter 9 for a vital signs recording sheet.

The following pages give details on how to measure each of the four vital signs, as well as what the values can mean.

General Tips for Measuring Vital Signs

It can be challenging to measure vital signs in a person with dementia. Here are some tips to make it easier:

- Try measuring all four vital signs one right after the other. Have everything handy before you start:
    - Pencil and paper to write down the measurements
    - A watch or clock with a second hand
    - A digital thermometer with the tip cleaned
    - A blood pressure machine (if you have one)
- Vital signs are affected by mood and physical activity. To get the most accurate readings:
    - Wait until the person seems calm. It may help to give them something to hold, a show to watch, or music to listen to.
    - Help the person to sit comfortably, waiting at least 10 minutes after physical activity.
- You can often check the pulse and breathing rate without the person knowing you're doing it.

Alzheimer's Medical Advisor provides online instructional videos on vital sign measurement, pain, dehydration, and more. View these videos at alzmed.unc.edu/videos.

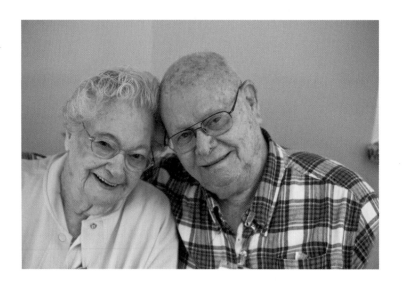

- For temperature and blood pressure, you'll need to use equipment. For these measurements, give simple directions and explain what you're going to do before doing it.

- If you get an unusual reading and the person seems okay, wait 10-20 minutes and measure again.

- If the person gets upset, give them space and try again later.

Examples of times when measuring vital signs can be helpful:

- When the person is healthy, to know the person's normal or usual range

- After a fall or injury

- If you're worried about dehydration

- If the person has a sudden change in their behavior (for example, agitated, aggressive, sleepy, or weak)

- If you think the person may be in pain

- If the person has a new medical symptom like cough, diarrhea, or rash

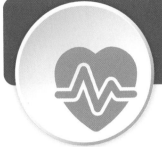

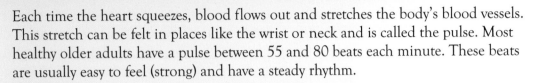

Pulse

Each time the heart squeezes, blood flows out and stretches the body's blood vessels. This stretch can be felt in places like the wrist or neck and is called the pulse. Most healthy older adults have a pulse between 55 and 80 beats each minute. These beats are usually easy to feel (strong) and have a steady rhythm.

Low Pulse

Pulses below 55 beats per minute are usually considered low, although it may be normal for someone taking certain blood pressure medicines. Low pulse can be caused by a problem with the heart, thyroid or other organs.

High Pulse

A pulse above 80 beats per minute when the person is resting is a bit high but can be normal; pulses over 100 are abnormal. Pain, anxiety, fever, blood loss, dehydration and heart problems can cause high pulse.

Weak or Irregular Pulse

Pulses that are unusually weak or hard to find, or that don't have a steady rhythm, can also be signs of a problem. Certain heart conditions, like atrial fibrillation, cause the pulse to be irregular and weak. By checking the person's pulse often, you'll be tuned into any changes from usual.

Low, high, weak or irregular pulse can be an emergency, especially if the person also has any of these:

- Trouble breathing
- Chest pain
- Passing out
- Falls
- Dizziness
- Worsening confusion
- Weakness

How to Measure Pulse

1. Get a piece of paper, pen or pencil, and a watch or clock with a second hand. Have the person seated and as relaxed as possible.

2. Lay the person's arm palm side up and use your index and middle fingertips to find the pulse on the wrist, just under the thumb. It may help to ask first if you can hold hands.

3. If you don't feel it right away, try slightly different areas on the wrist and different amounts of pressure. If you're still having trouble, try feeling the other wrist.

4. Count the pulse for one minute, paying attention to the rhythm and strength.

5. Write the number down.

Pulse
Typical low, normal and high heart beats per minute. Exact ranges vary by person.

Low	Normal				High	
30	40	50	60	70	80	90	100	110

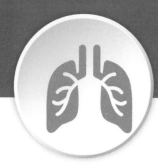

Breathing Rate

Breathing rate is the number of breaths a person takes in one minute. Most healthy older adults take between 10 and 20 breaths each minute at rest. People with chronic lung diseases, like COPD, may have a higher "normal" breathing rate.

Low Breathing Rate

Breathing rates below 10 breaths per minute are usually considered low, although they may be normal if the person is sleeping or very relaxed. Low breathing rates can be caused by too much medication or a brain problem (like a previous stroke).

High Breathing Rate

Breathing rates above 20 breaths per minute are usually considered high, and rates over 25 are usually a sign of illness. Severe pain, anxiety, or problems with the heart or lungs can cause high breathing rates. Fast breathing is a common sign of pneumonia.

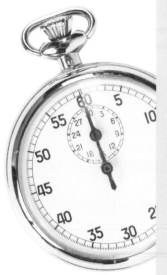

High breathing rates can be an emergency, especially if one or more of these is present:

- Has bluish lips, fingers or fingertips
- Has chest pain
- Has trouble talking at rest
- Can't lie flat
- Is straining their neck muscles while breathing
- Has wheezing or noisy breathing

How to Measure the Breathing Rate

1 Get a piece of paper, pen or pencil, and a watch or clock with a second hand. Have the person seated and as relaxed as possible.

2 Count the number of times the person breathes both in and out for one minute. Each time the chest and shoulders move up and down counts as one breath. If needed, touch their shoulder lightly to feel the breaths.

3 Write down the number.

Tip: Don't tell the person you're measuring their breathing, or they may start to breathe differently.

Breathing Rate

Typical low, normal and high breaths per minute. Exact ranges vary by person.

Low	Normal		High	
5	10	15	20	25	30

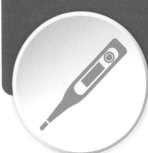

Body Temperature

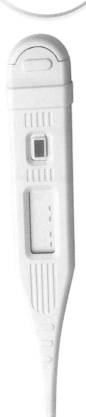

Older persons tend to have lower body temperatures. For many, readings in the 97° F range are typical, with variations depending on the time of day taken (temperatures are lowest in the morning and highest in the evening). Also, rectal and ear temperatures tend to be a little higher than oral, while under arm measurements are a bit lower. It's important to know the person's usual readings at different times of day, so that you'll be alert to changes.

Low Body Temperature

If you measure an unusually low body temperature and the person seems okay, try giving the person a blanket or sweater and measure again later. If the person seems ill, contact their provider.

High Body Temperature (Fever)

In general, a reading 1.2° F or more above the person's usual temperature for that time of day is considered a fever. Often, readings over 99° F by mouth are high, and readings over 100.5° F may be serious. Fever is most often caused by infections in the respiratory tract (like bronchitis or pneumonia), urinary tract, or skin.

How to Measure Body Temperature

1 Get a piece of paper, pen or pencil, and digital thermometer with a tip that's been washed in room temperature soapy water and dried.

2 To take a temperature by mouth: Turn the thermometer on and place it under one side of the tongue and towards the back of the mouth. *Tip: Make sure the person doesn't talk, bite down, or breathe through their mouth.*

3 To take a temperature under the arm: Turn the thermometer on, lift the arm, and place the tip under the arm against the skin. Lower the arm and hold it gently in place. *Tip: Make sure the tip stays under the arm, and isn't sticking out the back.*

4 When the thermometer beeps, take it out, read the temperature, and write the number down.

Fever can be an emergency, especially if the person:

- Has fever over 101° F
- Has signs of delirium (page 48)
- Has trouble breathing

See page 70 for more on fever

Temperature

Typical low, normal and high body temperature ranges by mouth.
Exact ranges vary by person.

Low		Normal			High		
95°	96°	97°	98°	99°	100°	101°	102°

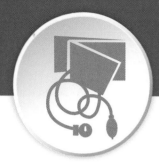

Blood Pressure

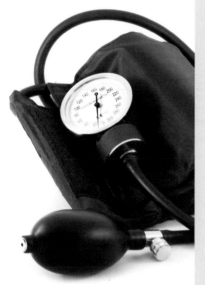

Blood pressure measurements include two numbers. The higher (systolic) number is the pressure as the heart squeezes blood out. The lower (diastolic) number is the pressure as the heart relaxes. Each person's blood pressure can vary depending on things like the time of day, medicines, caffeine, mood, and physical activity. Record blood pressure during the morning, afternoon, and evening for a few days to find the normal range.

Low Blood Pressure

What is considered "low" blood pressure depends on the person. For many, systolic readings less than 90 or diastolic readings less than 60 are low. Usually, low blood pressure isn't a problem unless the person feels faint or dizzy. Common causes include medications, dehydration, and viral illnesses (like the flu).

High Blood Pressure

If the person consistently has systolic pressure over 140 and/or diastolic pressure over 90 (or whatever level the person's primary care physician recommends, if different), notify the provider. If the person also has symptoms of a possible emergency (see box), get medical help right away, as it can mean a problem with the heart, kidneys, brain or other organs. For more information on high blood pressure see page 82.

LOW blood pressure can be an emergency if the person also has:

- Dizziness or fainting spells
- Signs of delirium (page 48) or dehydration (page 142)

HIGH blood pressure can be an emergency, especially if:

- You measure over 220 systolic and/or over 120 diastolic several times
- The person has chest pain (page 44), signs of a stroke (page 120), or trouble breathing (page 40)

How to Measure Blood Pressure Using a Machine

1 Help the person to sit comfortably and relax for at least five minutes before measuring.

2 Ask the person to sit with legs uncrossed and flat on the floor. Crossing the legs can raise the blood pressure by up to 10 points.

3 Ask the person to place their arm, palm up, at the height of their heart—for example, on an arm rest.

4 Wrap the cuff around the skin of the upper arm (not over clothing), two finger widths above the elbow. Have the arrow on the cuff point toward the bend in the elbow.

5 Follow the machine's instructions to read the blood pressure. When it's done, write down the result.

Tip: If you get a reading that is unusual, wait at least 10 minutes and take it again.

Be sure you're using the right size cuff. A regular cuff is fine for most people. People with very large arms need a large cuff; tiny arms need a small cuff.

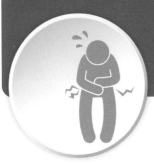

Pain

Recognizing and Preventing Pain

As we age, aches and pains become more common. Common causes of pain in older persons include arthritis, back or neck problems, muscle stiffness from not moving enough, intestinal problems like gas or constipation, swollen or sore feet, and problems with the teeth or gums.

Someone with dementia may not express pain in typical ways, and so it may go unnoticed and untreated. For example, they may use words like "tight" or "broken down" or just moan or groan. As dementia progresses, facial expressions, body movements, or behavior can be clues to pain. The person may not want to move a body part, may cover it, or get upset when touched. For example, if the person gets fidgety, withdraws, or kicks when you try to wash their feet, it's probably because their feet hurt.

If you're concerned about pain and the person can communicate, ask them about it with simple yes/no questions. Try gently touching the area of the body where you suspect pain while watching their reaction closely. If you think the person has pain, change what you're doing. If it persists, get medical attention.

Tips to Prevent and Treat Pain during Daily Care

- Plan daily care (like bathing or brushing teeth) at times when the person is most rested and relaxed.
- Give pain medicine 1–2 hours before starting a painful activity.
- Keep the room well-lit and at a comfortable temperature.
- Offer a distraction like calming music.
- Give simple directions.
- Say what you're going to do before you do it.
- If the person is upset or shows signs of pain, stop what you are doing, pause, and start again being more slow or gentle.

Common Signs of Pain in Persons with Dementia:

Words and Sounds:
- Words like "ache," "heavy," "ouch," "funny," "not right"
- Moaning
- Shouting out
- Noisy breathing
- Sighing, crying
- Whimpering

Facial Expressions:
- Grimacing
- Wrinkled nose
- Eyebrow furrowed
- Eyes shut tight
- Sad or scared
- Raised corner of mouth

Body Movements:
- Rigid, tense, still
- Covering, rubbing, shaking, or protecting a body part
- Changes in the way they walk or move

Behavior:
- Agitated, restless
- Aggressive, angry
- Withdrawn, not doing things they enjoy
- More confused
- Change in eating or sleeping
- Yelling
- Overreacting

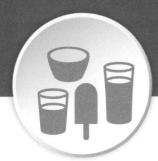

Dehydration

Recognizing and Preventing Dehydration

Dehydration is lower than normal fluid levels in the body caused by not drinking enough or losing too much fluid. Both situations are common in older persons with dementia. In fact, as the disease progresses, they commonly lose their sense of thirst, forget to drink, or have trouble asking for a drink. These problems are made worse if the person is sick, overheated, or takes medicines that dry them out.

By paying attention to how much fluid a person with dementia is drinking, caregivers can often catch problems early. If left untreated, dehydration can lead to problems like constipation, falls, worsening confusion or weakness, and even hospitalization.

If the person has one or more signs of dehydration and they're able to drink, use the tips on this page and watch them closely. If the person doesn't get better or if their signs are severe, seek medical help.

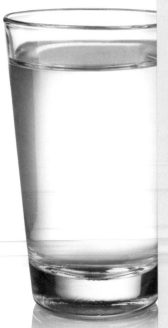

Tips to Prevent and Treat Dehydration

- Aim for 4 to 6 cups of fluid each day.
- Increase to 8 or more cups if the person is sick, overheated, or has signs of dehydration.
- Keep track of fluid intake daily to be sure it's enough.
- Offer choices—not just water. Try flavored water, juices, milk, smoothies, fruit, low-sodium soups, popsicles, sherbet, pudding or gelatin. Make sure the food or drink is at the temperature they like.
- Limit drinks that can be drying, such as those with caffeine and alcohol.
- Try different containers, such as sports bottles, sippy cups, straws, or small bottled waters. In advanced dementia, try a syringe.
- Keep drinks within reach and, if needed, remind the person how to lift the cup to their mouth and swallow.
- Offer drinks regularly throughout the day as part of the routine, not just with meals.
- Make drinking fun and social. Join them for an afternoon tea or non-alcoholic social hours.
- If you're concerned about nighttime incontinence, limit fluids in the 2–3 hours before bedtime and offer plenty of fluids throughout the day.
- If you're still having trouble, talk with a health care provider. See page 46 for trouble with swallowing, page 98 for more tips on not eating or drinking, and page 130 for tips on fluids when vomiting.

Common Signs of Dehydration:

- Dry eyes, nose and mouth
- Urinating less often or in smaller amounts than usual (especially going 8 or more hours without urination)
- Faster than usual heart rate (especially over 100 beats per minute)
- New or worsening weakness, confusion or sleepiness
- Weight loss

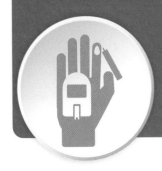

Diabetes and Other Chronic Illnesses

A person with dementia who has other chronic illnesses will need extra support to manage the illnesses. As a caregiver, it's important to work closely with health care providers to develop a care plan that works for your situation.

If you care for someone with dementia and **diabetes**:

- Talk with the health care provider about the goals of care. For example, hemoglobin AlC goals may be higher than typically recommended when tight control of blood sugar is difficult or unsafe.

- Ask about programs that connect families to nurses, pharmacists, nutritionists, or social workers with diabetes expertise. Take advantage of community resources and caregiver support groups in your area.

- Learn to recognize the symptoms of low and high blood sugar (page 61), keeping in mind that symptoms can sometimes be mistaken for dementia. If you're concerned, check the sugar. Keep high sugar foods handy in case of a low blood sugar emergency.

- For more tips on helping someone with diabetes, including tips for when the person resists care, see page 61.

Any chronic illness is more difficult when complicated by dementia. Here are some tips about other common chronic diseases:

- **In chronic lung disease,** dementia makes it especially difficult to coordinate the use of inhalers. If this is happening, ask the medical provider about a spacer or nebulizer device, which can make medication use easier.

- In persons with dementia who have **glaucoma or other eye problems**, caregivers should usually take over the administration of eye drops early on, as both coordination and memory losses make using them correctly difficult even early in the illness.

- In **any illness,** a key to success is to simplify the treatment plan. If the person is on medications twice a day, ask if they can be once a day. If the person is on many medications, ask which ones are most essential and which ones are less important.

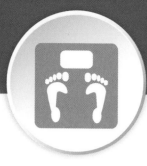

Nutrition and Weight

Under-nutrition—not taking in enough food to stay healthy—is common in persons with dementia. Over time, this can lead to weight loss. It also makes the person more likely to fall, get sick, heal slowly, and be less able to care for themselves. For these reasons, it's important to follow weight closely and troubleshoot early when problems arise. Unexpected weight loss of 5 or more pounds in a month should prompt a visit to the health care provider.

Less commonly, a person with dementia may become overweight from overeating. Sometimes this is because they don't remember that they've already eaten or they're worried about not having enough food. Persons with frontotemporal dementia may crave certain foods or eat things that aren't food. These cases can be particularly challenging and stressful for families.

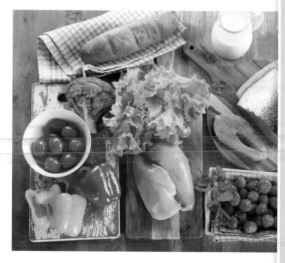

Tips for Healthy Eating

Diet recommendations for persons with dementia are the same as those for healthy older adults. Most experts agree that a diet rich in fruits, vegetables and whole grains, with moderate amounts of protein from dairy, fish and poultry will meet nutritional needs. However, be flexible and make foods appealing, even if it means a "less healthy" choice every now and then.

- Offer a variety of foods that the person enjoys, with easy-to-eat finger foods and high-energy snacks between meals.

- Tastes can change with aging. Try different foods and seasonings.

- If the person is losing weight and is on a restricted diet due to another condition, talk with their health care provider about allowing more flexibility.

- If the person is overweight, keep less healthy foods out of the home and offer activities to keep them busy between meals.

- If you are uncertain, ask a health care provider or nutritionist. They'll check for medical conditions and for deficiencies of certain vitamins, like B12 or folate.

- Over-the-counter nutritional drinks, when given in addition to usual meals and snacks, can help prevent weight loss and promote weight gain.

- For more tips on managing poor appetite and weight loss, see page 98 on not eating or drinking.

Tips for Making the Most of Mealtimes

Recent research has focused on ways to make family meals an enjoyable time of connection and companionship. It shows that if we pay more attention to socializing and relationships during meals instead of focusing on what and how the person is eating, the person may feel better, eat more, and eat more healthfully. Here are some strategies to try:

- Make meals an important ritual of the day, where family members eat together.

- Plan the menu together.

- Use mealtimes as a chance to talk about the day or reminisce. It's okay if the person just listens. Try talking about the food or what you see out the window. Consider reading letters from family or an interesting news article.

- Try to give the person your full attention without distractions.

- When possible, use humor and be easygoing.

- Try to focus on strengths while overlooking mistakes.

- Try to be flexible. What works or is interesting one day may not work the next.

- Recognize the importance of letting the person do for him or herself. Find a way to keep the person involved in the process of preparing, eating and cleaning up afterwards. Then, show appreciation for their help.

Nutrition in Advanced Dementia

As dementia progresses to an advanced stage, appetite loss, difficulties chewing and swallowing, and accompanying weight loss are normal and expected.

- Pressuring the person to eat or drink will be stressful for both you and them.

- Artificial feeding with a tube is uncomfortable, has side effects, and is not recommended in advanced dementia.

- If the person is near the end of life, offer frequent small amounts of "comfort food" such as ice cream, and sips of a favorite drink. Keep the mouth moist using a swab or cloth. Usually, this is enough to satisfy any hunger or thirst the person feels.

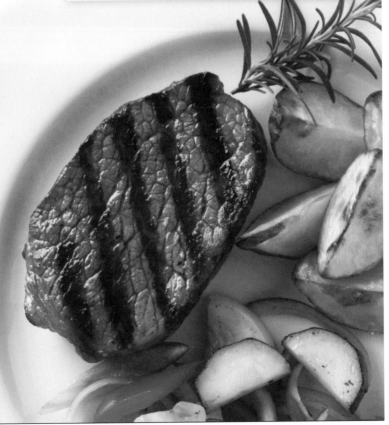

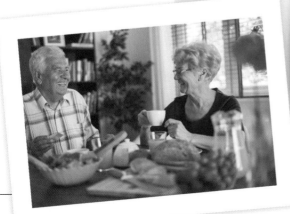

> When it's time for Mom to take her medicine, the less I say, the better it goes. I just hand her one pill at a time and a small cup of water. It's easier if I don't try to explain everything.
>
> *— Dorothy S., caregiver*

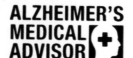

Medication Safety and Management

Managing medications for a person with dementia can be a tough challenge for family caregivers. Caregivers must understand the reason for, use of, and common side effects of specific medications; make sure the person with dementia is taking their medication correctly and safely; make sure the person is not secretly self-medicating; and monitor for the desired effects and potential side effects. Typically a family caregiver has to:

- Read the medication label and understand what the medication is for and its directions for use.
- Make sure each medication is necessary and the dose is right. The person's health care provider should review the medication list about every 6 to 12 months. By stopping unnecessary medications or changing a dose, the person with dementia may be able to take medications less often with fewer side effects.
- Keep an up-to-date list of all medications in an easy to find place (like the refrigerator). Be sure this list includes the name of all medications (prescriptions, vitamins, herbals, supplements), the dose, and how and when it is taken. At the end of this book you'll find a sheet you can use to list medications and health information.
- Understand the risks, benefits, and potential side effects of each new medication.
- Make sure the person is taking the right medicine at the right time and gets their medication refilled.
- Watch for side effects.
- Understand the risks of medication interactions with foods, supplements, and non-prescription medications.

Start low and go slow when starting a medication is a principle that applies to all older persons and especially to persons with dementia. Older persons tend to be more sensitive to medications and so often need less than a young adult. Starting with a low dose helps identify side effects when they are not too severe.

There are several types of medications that can be used to help prevent or treat medical problems.

- **Prescribed medications** must be prescribed by a health care provider such as a medical doctor or nurse practitioner. Typically the prescription is given to a pharmacist in a drug store, but you can sometimes order medications by mail. Prescription medications can either come as brand-name or generic. A **brand-name** medication has a patent and so is typically more costly and available from only one drug company; a **generic** medication has been available for a longer period of time and is often less expensive.

- **Over-the-counter** medications can be purchased without a prescription. These medications are typically bought in a drug store or pharmacy. Examples include cough medicine, antacids, or pain medication such as acetaminophen (Tylenol). Over-the-counter medications can be as harmful in combination with prescription medicines, though, so it's important to read the bottle carefully and follow the directions.

- **Supplements and herbal medications** may also interact with other medications, so it's important to tell the person's health care provider and pharmacist which supplements and herbal remedies the person is taking, and in what dose. If a person with dementia is having trouble taking a supplement or herbal medication, consider if there are alternative ways to accomplish the same goal, such as eating healthy foods or drinking more calcium rich foods.

Medications come in different forms. The next pages provide information about the types of medications and things to consider about each.

Medication Forms Designed to Be Swallowed or Dissolved in the Mouth

Medication Type		Description	Things to Know
Tablet		Powdered medication compressed into hard disk or cylinder	• If a tablet has a line through the middle, it may be broken to give smaller doses; it's okay to crush it into a powder.
Caplet		Solid pill shaped like a capsule and coated for ease of swallowing	• Similar to tablets except for the shape. Most can be crushed.
Enteric coated tablet or caplet		Tablet that is coated so it won't dissolve in the stomach	• Coating eases stomach upset. Do not crush—it destroys the coating.
Capsule		Medication encased in a gelatin shell	• Usually has a liquid or small pellets in it. You may be able to open the capsule and sprinkle pellets in food or liquid. If the person won't swallow it, ask about a liquid version.
Lozenge		Flat, candy-like, round pill that dissolves in the mouth	• Designed to dissolve in the mouth rather than being swallowed.
Syrup		Medication dissolved in a concentrated sweet liquid	• Must be measured with a measuring cup, syringe or spoon.

If Someone with Dementia Refuses or Has Trouble Swallowing Tablets, Capsules, or Caplets

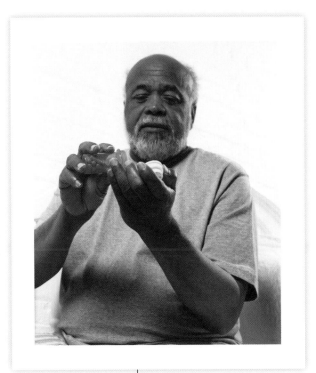

- Talk to the person's medical care provider about which medications are most important and whether some can be stopped.

- The person may suffer from a dry mouth. Try having them swallow water, juice, or coffee first and see if that helps them swallow their pill.

- The person may not recognize that the pill in their mouth is medication and needs to be swallowed. If so, ask their health care provider or pharmacist if the medication comes in liquid form (about 1/3 of medications do). Other options include dissolvable tablets or a transdermal patch.

- If none of these options work and one or more medications is absolutely necessary, see if it can be crushed and mixed with food.

Crushing Pills and Mixing Them with Food

If the person with dementia refuses to take pills or has trouble swallowing, and a medication does not come in liquid form, you may want to consider crushing their pills. If so, here are some things to know:

- Most tablets and caplets can be crushed; but extended release, timed release, or enteric coated medications should **not** be crushed. If you aren't sure, ask your pharmacist.

- A pill crusher can be purchased at a drug store. You can also use a mortar and pestle or place the pill in a sandwich bag and hit it with a hammer.

- Once you crush the pill into a powder, mix the powder in a **small** amount of applesauce, pudding, or yogurt (so the person will take the whole thing).

- Many pills are bitter; if so, the person may not want to take it unless the food you mix it with can disguise the flavor.

- If the person has early dementia and is suspicious or paranoid but generally aware of what's going on, think twice about crushing pills—you may have more of a problem if they find out.

Medications Placed On or Rubbed Into the Skin, Inside of the Nose, or Vagina

Type	Description	Example(s)	Things to Know
Ointment	Greasy medication for application on the skin	A&D ointment; vaseline	• Leaves a greasy surface that helps prevent drying. • Typically does not absorb well into the skin, so it is most commonly used in the eye or nose.
Paste	Similar to ointment, but thicker	Zinc oxide paste	• Absorbs through the skin more slowly than ointment. • Wear gloves when applying it. • For use on the outside of the body only.
Cream	Medication is dissolved in a thick cream	Hydrocortisone cream	• Used only on the skin or in the vagina. • Often can be rubbed in, not leaving as greasy a surface as ointments and pastes.
Transdermal patch	Disk or patch containing medication; the drug is absorbed through the skin	Patches for nicotine, pain medication, or Exelon (for brain function)	• Usually meant to stay on for 1-3 days. • Placed on the skin, it provides medication that goes throughout the body. • Change patch per instructions. • Be sure to remove the old patch before applying a new one. • Watch for skin rash (reaction) at the site.

Tips on Administering an Ointment, Paste or Cream

- Remember this is a medication and you do not want to get it on your skin. Wear gloves if you need to rub the ointment, paste, or cream on the skin.

- Gently clean the area with soap and water to remove the previously applied medication. Applying new medication over old medication can make it less effective.

- Watch out for skin irritation at the site where you apply the ointment, paste, or cream.

Tips on Applying a Transdermal Patch

- Follow the directions on the medication.

- When you remove the old patch, be gentle. Older skin can be fragile and it can be injured by stickiness of the patch.

- Do not touch the medicated surface of a patch—you may absorb some of the medication.

- To avoid skin irritation do not place a new transdermal patch on the same body part as the previous one.

Other Medication Types

Type	Description	Key Points
Suppository	Solid dosage mixed with gelatin and shaped in the form of a pellet for insertion into a body cavity (rectum or vagina)	• For rectal or vaginal use only. • Do not swallow. • Handle carefully, as it can melt in your hand. If it is soft, refrigerate before using. • Wear a glove when inserting the medication. • Lubricate the tip with lubricating jelly like K-Y jelly.
Inhaler	Inhaler is a portable, handheld device that delivers medication as a spray	• Follow the directions on the outside of the device. • If directions say to do so, shake the inhaler before using. • Press the inhaler while the person inhales. • Use a spacer (see description below) to help the spray get to the lungs.
Eye drops	Liquid meant to be placed into the eye using a dropper	• If you have trouble inserting the drops, an eye drop aid (dispenser) can be purchased at a drug store. • Do not touch the tip of the dropper to the eye; it can cause bacteria to go onto the dropper and can injure the person's eye.

Tips for Caregivers on Using Eye Drops

- Wash your hands before and after helping with eye drops.
- Have the person lie down on their back comfortably with a pillow under their head.
- Gently pull down the lower eyelid. Place one drop of the medication in the pocket of their lower lid.
- Do not touch the dropper to the eye.
- If you have trouble, get an eye drop aid or dispenser from a drug store.
- Steady the dropper so you will not accidentally touch it to the person's eye.

Tips for Caregivers on Insulin Injection

- If the person is agitated, wait until they are calm. Try an activity such as watching television to distract the person. Be sure you are both sitting down.
- Then calmly tell them that you will be giving them an injection.
- If the person with dementia is still resisting the injection, talk to their health care provider. It may be possible to provide a non-injectable alternative to the medication, or you might be able to get a nurse to come to the house and help.

Tips for Caregivers on Inhaler Use

- Use calm and simple directions. "This is your inhaler that helps you breathe. Put your mouth on it. Take a deep breath."
- If the problem is coordinating the timing of a deep breath with the puff of medication, try pressing the inhaler yourself as the person starts breathing in.
- If timing remains a problem, ask the pharmacist for a spacer—a tube you attach to the inhaler that the user puts their mouth on. When you press the inhaler, the medication gathers in the tube until the person takes a breath.
- If problems persist coordinating use of an inhaler, talk to the person's health care provider about using a nebulizer. A nebulizer is a machine that turns the medication into a mist that is then breathed in through a mask. The person can either wear the mask or you can hold the mask near their nose and mouth.

Medication Side Effects

Whenever a new medication is started, it's important to watch for side effects. Common side effects include nausea, vomiting, diarrhea, headache, fatigue, dizziness, and increased confusion. Some side effects tend to improve as time goes on; others may get worse. If a side effect is severe enough to affect function (such as balance or food intake) or doesn't improve within a few days, stop the medication and immediately contact the person's health care provider.

Medications with particularly frequent side effects include:

- **Non-steroidal anti-inflammatory drugs (NSAIDs) such as ibuprofen (Motrin or Advil), naproxen (Aleve), and others.** These are commonly used for pain. However, they can cause stomach upset, ulcers, intestinal bleeding, kidney problems, and leg swelling, especially with longstanding use and in older persons. Often acetaminophen (Tylenol) is a safer alternative.

- **Anti-anxiety drugs such as diazepam (Valium), lorazepam (Ativan) or alprazolam (Xanax).** These can cause confusion, drowsiness, trouble with balance, and falls. They should only be used as a last resort.

- **Anticholinergic drugs such as diphenhydramine (Benadryl), oxybutynin (Ditropan), codeine, or the Parkinson's drug trihexyphenidyl (Artane).** These often cause constipation, dry mouth, inability to urinate, confusion, and hallucinations.

- **Diabetes drugs such as glyburide (Micronase) or insulin.** If the dose is incorrect or the person has not eaten, these drugs can cause low blood sugar, which can lead to dizziness, falling, loss of consciousness, and coma.

- **Narcotic pain medications** such as morphine, Percocet, or oxycontin can cause dizziness, worsening confusion, sleepiness, falls, and constipation. They can be addictive and should be used only for short periods of time if possible.

- **Sleep medications** such as zolpidem (Ambien) are risky for people with dementia and can cause falls, confusion, and decreased self-care. They should only be used the a last resort. Sometimes a health care provider may prescribe the anti-depressant trazodone (Desaryl) to help with sleep. If these medications are prescribed, they should only be used for a short period of time. Also, the health care provider should provide the lowest dose possible. **Do not use sleep, pain, or anxiety medications if the person consumes alcohol.**

Side Effect versus Allergy

A **side effect** is an unwanted effect of a medication such as nausea, diarrhea, or tiredness. Most drugs have both desired effects and side effects, with the side effects varying from person to person. For example, a medication could affect the vomiting center in the brain, causing very mild nausea in one person and severe vomiting in another.

An **allergic reaction** is when the person's body reacts to a medication, leading to such things as hives, itching, face swelling, or trouble breathing. The culprit is the body's immune system. Allergic reactions are particularly dangerous because they can get bad fast. **If a person started a new medication and has difficulty breathing or swallowing, call 911 or go to the nearest emergency room.**

Medications Used to Improve Brain Function in Dementia

Unfortunately, we do not yet have many medication options to improve brain function in persons with Alzheimer's disease and other dementias, and the ones we have are by no means miracle cures. Still, in a few cases these drugs may improve attention or thinking.

Cholinesterase inhibitors such as donepezil (Aricept), rivastigmine (Exelon), and galantamine (Razadyne) are the medications most commonly used to treat memory loss associated with Alzheimer's disease. They are typically prescribed in the early to moderate stages and help to delay or keep memory loss from getting worse for a period of time. Common side effects include nausea, vomiting, poor appetite, and diarrhea.

Memantine (Namenda) is a medication to treat moderate to severe stages of Alzheimer's disease. This drug helps people with dementia keep their daily function, such as being able to use the bathroom without help. The side effects for Namenda include headache, constipation, confusion, and dizziness.

When **starting and stopping** these medications, most doctors like to start with a low dose and slowly increase it if the person is able to tolerate it without side effects. If the person has intolerable side effects or has been taking the medication for 3 to 6 months without any meaningful change in memory or behavior, you may want to consider stopping the medication. Ask yourself—is the person doing anything different in the past 3 months? What, if anything, has improved? If the answer is no, you may want to consider stopping the medication. If so, don't stop the drug suddenly. Instead, gradually reduce the dose over the course of a few weeks, as directed by a health care provider.

A hard decision for many is whether and when to stop one of these medications if the person has been on it for a long time. A common worry is that the person will suddenly get much worse; however, this rarely happens. This is a decision you'll want to make in consultation with a health care provider who knows the person with dementia well.

There are a fair number of dietary supplements and "medical foods" available over-the-counter that claim to improve brain function. However, safety, effectiveness, and purity standards are not as high for dietary supplements as they are for prescription drugs. There is also the potential for supplements to interact with prescription drugs. For this reason, it is important to discuss any decision to take a supplement with a trusted health care provider.

Medications Used to Control Agitation, Aggression or Other Behavioral Symptoms

Caregivers are often challenged by behaviors associated with dementia. These behaviors can include mood changes, wandering, hoarding or searching, hallucinations (seeing, hearing or feeling things that aren't there), delusions (unchangeable false thoughts), agitation, argumentativeness, false accusations, angry outbursts, inappropriate sexual behavior, resisting care, and striking out at others.

Experts agree that medications are NOT the preferred method of addressing these behaviors. Instead, what works best is changing the environment, activities, communication and interactions with the person living with dementia. Most "difficult" behaviors are reactions to something the person with dementia has experienced or an inability to describe unmet needs. For information about non-medication strategies, see our sections on agitation (page 30), aggression (page 32), hallucinations and delusions (page 74), hoarding or hiding things (page 86), resisting care (page 110), and sexual behavior (page 112).

In very difficult situations, health professionals will sometimes recommend a trial of a medication. Four types of medications are sometimes used:

- **Antipsychotic medications** such as haloperidol (Haldol), quetiapine (Seroquel), or risperidone (Risperdal). These medications need to be used with extreme caution because they are associated with sedation, falls, stroke and death when used by older people with dementia. Given this risk, the Food and Drug Administration states that they should only be used if (a) the behavior is related to psychosis, (b) the person is a danger to themselves or others, or (c) the person is so inconsolable that they cannot eat or drink because of distress. They should not be used to sedate or restrain a person with dementia. If used, it should be for a short period of time and the person should be closely monitored by a health care provider. Additionally, many antipsychotic medications are usually not advised in persons with Lewy body dementia, as they can cause severe reactions.

- **Non-antipsychotic tranquilizers** such as alprazolam (Xanax) or buspirone (Buspar). These drugs are sometimes used in small doses for anxiety or agitation. Side effects include making the person more confused, increasing the likelihood of falls, and in some cases reducing impulse control.

- **Medications used to improve brain function**. These were discussed on the previous page. Occasionally, if a person is not already on one of these medications, introducing the medication will lead to an improvement in behavioral symptoms. Unfortunately, in some cases, the opposite happens.

- **Antidepressant medications.** These are often used to treat depression, anxiety, low mood, and irritability in people with dementia; examples include citalopram (Celexa), escitalopram (Lexapro), sertraline (Zoloft), and trazodone (Desyrel). These medications are occasionally helpful in persons with depression who appear depressed; however, they are less effective in dementia in younger adults. There also is some evidence that citalopram may help with aggression and agitation behaviors; however, this medication has been linked to heart disease and poorer performance on memory tests, so the risks and benefits should be considered before use.

Managing Medications as Dementia Progresses

Medication management is one of the main reasons why persons with dementia move into assisted living or a nursing home setting. This means that a family caregiver's attention to medication management is a key factor in keeping someone with dementia at home. How you get involved in medication management will depend on the severity of the dementia and the person's individual needs.

In the **early stages of dementia**, when the person is accustomed to managing their own medication, a common issue involves whether they are taking their medicines safely. This can be challenging because the person may want to continue managing their medicines themselves. Here are some tips on helping someone in early dementia take their medications independently and safely:

- Use a pill organizer box that you fill up once a week, and store the bottles of labeled medications somewhere safe. If the person takes medicines more than once a day, use a box that has compartments labeled "AM" and "PM."

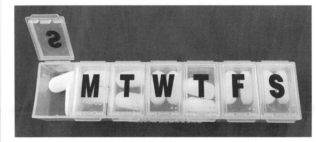

- Create a routine to help the person remember to take their medications. If the medication is typically taken at breakfast, put the pill box next to the coffee maker. If taken before bed, place the pill box next to the person's toothbrush.

- Try to fit the medication schedule to the person's daily routine. Some people sleep late; others change their sleep pattern in other ways.

- Use reminders such as an alarm or a daily phone call to help the person remember their medication when you can't be there.

- If you believe the person is no longer able to take their medication safely, try to enlist them in working together with you. Say something like "How about if we work as a team to be sure you're safe in managing all these medications."

- Self medicating and refusals are quite common in early stages because the person gets fixed on one medical condition and/or doesn't accept need for treatment of another condition like dementia.

In **later stages of dementia** the caregiver will need to take on full responsibility for giving the person their medications. Here are some guidelines for doing this successfully:

- Ask the health care provider or pharmacist to simplify the medication list. It may be possible to reduce the number of medications and/or the number of times a day the person takes medication.

- When giving medication, use simple, clear language. For example, say "Here is the pill for your arthritis pain, put it in your mouth." Hand them a glass of water and say "Have a drink of water to help the pill go down."

- If the person refuses to take medication, don't argue or fight. Instead, stop and try to find out why. They may have mouth pain; the medication may taste bad; or they may not remember how to swallow a pill or what it's for. Explain simply. It may help to remind the person that "this is the pill you requested for your pain" or that someone they trust (such as their doctor or son) thinks it will really help. If they continue to refuse, try again later.

- If the person repeatedly refuses to take medication, ask their health care provider to make sure that there isn't a physical cause for the refusal. They also may identify an easier way to give the medication, such as in a liquid or dissolvable tablet.

- For safety, keep all medications in a locked drawer or cabinet.

- If you can't be present at medication time, arrange for someone else to help.

Common Medication Management Questions

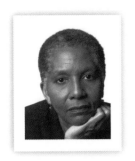

"My dad insists on managing his own medicines, and I'm afraid he's making mistakes. What can I do?"

Clues that medication management is not going well include not getting refills on schedule, finding pills left over when they should have run out, needing a refill before it's due, and potential side effects such as increased confusion, dizziness, or falling. If the person is forgetting to take medications their health may suffer; for example, blood pressure may be high or blood sugar less well controlled.

The best way to ensure the person is taking their medication properly is for someone to watch them take the medication. If that's not possible, then work with him around having a reminder system, using such things as a pill box in a convenient place that you fill weekly, an alarm clock (or pill box with a built-in alarm), or a phone call daily that includes asking about their medication.

If you're worried that the person is taking too much medication, has stopped taking it, or is taking another medication on their own, notify their health care provider.

"My husband missed a dose of his medicine. What should I do?"

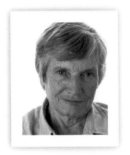

For most medications, missing a dose will have little health impact. Generally it's best to take the next dose at the normal time and in the normal amount. Doubling up more than doubles the risk of a side effect. AVOID DOUBLE DOSES. If your husband misses medications frequently, discuss it with the health care provider.

"I help mom with her medication, and lately she's been refusing to take her pills. It's so frustrating."

If the person with dementia is refusing to take their medications, try to figure out why. Is something bothering them, like a toothache or sore throat? Is there something about the way you approach her that is making her feel anxious or pressured? Does she not understand what the pill is for, or perhaps even who you are? Does one or more of her pills taste bitter? Has she gagged or nearly gagged on a pill recently? When the pill is in her mouth, does she forget what it is?

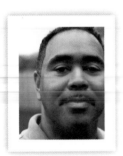

In addition to trying to address any specific problem you identify, here are some general tips:

- Provide a calm environment, and be calm and patient.
- Guide her through the process and encourage her to do as much as she can and wants. If she can't open the pill bottle, perhaps she can pick the pill up herself.
- If she gets upset, take a break and try again later.
- If your frustration is making the problem worse, see if someone else can help and/or talk to a health professional about what you can do.

You might try gentle encouragement like:

- "You told me you always feel better after you take it."
- "You asked me to remind you to take the medicine for your back pain" (or whatever symptom is prominent in their minds).

"When my mother's doctor prescribes a new medication, what questions should I ask about it?"

When a health care provider prescribes a new medication, here are some questions you should ask:

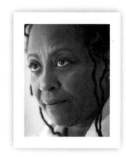

- What is the name of the medication, and does it go by another name?
- Why is this medication being prescribed?
- Is it necessary that the person take this medication? Are there any alternatives?
- How often and at what time of day should the medication be taken?
- Can the medication be taken with food, or should it be taken on an empty stomach?
- Are there any side effects that I should watch for?
- How much does this medication cost? Are there less costly or free alternatives (see below).

"My wife's medications are so expensive; we can't even afford the co-pay. What can we do?"

If you can't afford a medication, talk to the person's health care provider. A generic version of the medication or a less expensive alternative may be available. It also may be helpful to talk with a social worker because there may be programs available to help with medication costs.

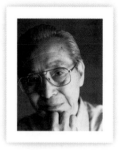

"My mom takes insulin because of diabetes. Now that she has dementia, what should I do?"

Insulin can be difficult to manage in someone with dementia, especially if the person wants to be involved. Not only are vision problems common in many older persons, but judgment and precision often suffer even early in dementia. Ways to prevent problems include pre-filled syringes, an injection pen, or getting off insulin entirely. If your mom is used to managing her own diabetes, get involved and learn how it should be done. A nurse in your mother's medical office can teach you how to test blood sugar, manage high and low blood sugar, and give insulin shots.

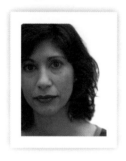

"My dad is used to drinking wine, beer or cocktails in the evenings, and he's on seven medications. Is this a problem?"

Many medications have side effects that can be worsened with alcohol, especially if the medication has side effects such as dizziness, drowsiness, or trouble with balance. Anti-anxiety, anti-psychotic, and sleeping medications are particularly likely to cause problems with alcohol. In addition, many other medications will have their effect altered by alcohol; so, it's important to read the information that comes with a drug.

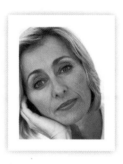

If your dad consumes alcohol as part of his routine, you'll need to decide whether the risk of a drug interaction is more or less important than the enjoyment (and, in many cases, appetite stimulation), provided by the alcohol. If you are especially concerned, consider buying non-alcoholic wine, beer, or spirits, maybe even joining him with a "drink" when you are able.

"When my husband was in the hospital, I put on a lot of music. It helped provide an environment I hoped he found supportive.

— *Kathy L., caregiver*

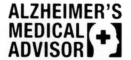

Health Care System

Throughout the course of illness, persons with dementia often require services from multiple types of health care providers in many different settings. Navigating the health care system can be overwhelming for both the caregiver and the person they care for—particularly when care is urgent, unexpected, or brings change to routines.

Use this chapter to guide you on how to make the most of the services available, including what questions to ask, answers to common caregiver concerns, and tips for decreasing the stress that often accompanies these encounters.

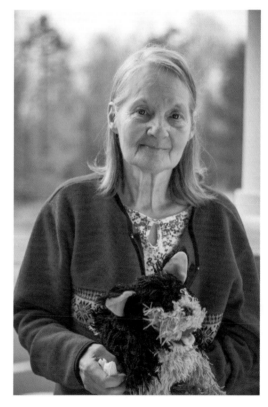

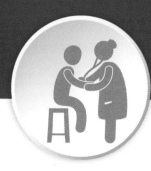

Primary Care Provider

What is a Primary Care Provider?

A primary care provider (PCP) is an important part of the care team for a person with dementia. It's the PCP who gets to know a person's general health, provides routine check-ups, and gets called when a person is sick. A PCP may be a family physician, a general internist, a nurse practitioner, or a physician's assistant.

Why a Person Needs a Primary Care Provider

- PCPs provide care over a long period of time, for a variety of health problems, and therefore become particularly familiar with the person. If the person with dementia is in a familiar place with familiar people, they are less likely to become confused and agitated.

- PCPs keep track of all the health problems a person has. They can coordinate treatments and medications for all of the person's health concerns, not just dementia.

- Because they are familiar with the person's overall health, PCPs can diagnose new problems and are often in the best position (other than family) to notice changes in a person with dementia. They can also recommend specialists they trust, if necessary.

- It is often easier to visit with a PCP than a specialist. Also, your PCP or their nurse will be the best person to call when you have concerns about the person's condition.

- Often the PCP can provide or help coordinate care for someone in the hospital. After a person is hospitalized, their health care needs may change. The PCP can help the caregiver and the person with dementia once the person is out of the hospital.

- PCPs can help from the time of dementia diagnosis through the end-of-life stage. If the person with dementia moves to a nursing home, sometimes the PCP will provide care there, too.

During Your Appointment

- Choose a time of day that both you and the person with dementia are comfortable with. Try not to schedule an appointment during meal or sleep times.

- To prevent the person with dementia from getting agitated, bring snacks and activities to distract them.

- Make sure to schedule follow up appointments.

How to Request Private Time with the PCP:

Sometimes, especially in earlier dementia stages, caregivers are unable to talk freely while the person with dementia is in the room. In this case, it's important to find a way to speak privately.

Consider e-mailing the PCP in advance, or discretely pass a note during the visit that explains the situation. Say something like "I have some questions I'd like to discuss but am concerned about upsetting [the person]. Can you arrange for us to speak privately?"

Things to Consider When Choosing a Primary Care Provider

- Pick a location that is easy to get to.

- Find an office that is open at times that are convenient to you.

- Choose a place where it is easy to get an appointment.

- Try to find a PCP experienced in dementia care. One way to do this is to ask a member of a dementia support group for their recommendations.

- Choose a provider who explains health issues clearly, including the diagnosis, the treatment plan, and what to expect.

- Find a provider who is willing and able to answer questions.

- Make sure the provider spends enough time with you and the person with dementia during the appointment.

- Choose a place where the provider or a nurse respond to your phone calls promptly.

- If it's difficult to drive the person with dementia from place to place, look for a PCP whose office draws blood and takes x-rays.

- Be sure to visit a new provider before the person with dementia gets sick.

What if you like your current primary care provider but find that they don't know much about dementia?

If your primary care provider doesn't provide helpful answers to your questions about dementia, consider also seeing a dementia specialist such as a geriatrician, neurologist, or geriatric nurse specialist.

Don't be afraid to change providers if you are not comfortable with the person's current provider.

If you decide to change providers:

- Make sure you have the new PCP lined up before telling your current primary care provider.

- Get copies of the person's medical record and current medications to give to the new provider.

- When making the appointment with the new provider, tell them the person is a new patient.

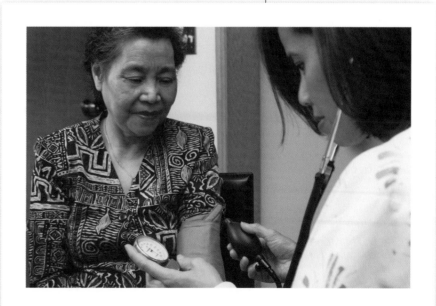

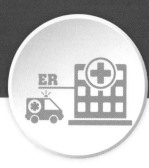

Emergency Care

Emergency Services Include:

- **Ambulance services**—Available in all communities. Medicare pays 80% if an emergency; if not an emergency, Medicare may refuse to pay.

- **Hospital emergency departments**—Places with lots of personnel and medical equipment for treating urgent problems such as heart attacks, strokes, seizures, broken bones, and serious mental health problems. They also care for a wide range of chronic and less serious problems, such as sore throats and chronic back pain, especially at night, weekends or holidays. However, they tend to be slow, noisy, chaotic, and expensive; so, they are best avoided except in true emergencies.

- Payment is generally covered by Medicare, with the person or their co-insurance required to pay 20% of the Medicare-approved amount, after they've met the yearly Part B deductible.

- For a person with dementia, a trip to the emergency department can be unpleasant and may be hazardous. Therefore, someone should always accompany a person with dementia.

- **How Emergency Departments Are Organized.** No appointment is needed. Patients can either arrive via ambulance or their own transportation. When a patients arrives, a nurse checks their vital signs, assesses their condition, and assigns a priority level. Patients with potentially life-threatening illnesses or injuries are seen immediately; others will often have to wait. After treatment, patients either go home or to the hospital for further treatment.

Common Caregiver Concerns around Emergency Department Visits—What You Can Do

Concern	What You Can Do
Getting there	• Don't hesitate to call 911 for an ambulance if transport by car is difficult.
Noise and commotion	• Ask if there's a quiet area where the patient can wait. • Bring music and/or noise cancelling headphones. • Bring activities to distract the person (such as a favorite movie).
Communication problems	• Explain the person's condition. • Ask staff to speak slowly and distinctly. • Explain whether the patient's mental state is the same or different.
Long waiting times	• Bring snacks and drinks. • Locate the nearest bathroom and take the person there periodically.
Complications from the visit or the treatment	• Ask questions. Ask what any test or medication is for, whether it is necessary, and what the side effects might be. • If staff want to put in a urinary catheter, ask if it's really necessary. • If the person gets agitated or more confused, stay with them, hold their hand, and talk with them. For more on delirium treatment, see page 48.

Checklist of Things to Bring to the Emergency Department

☐ Your cell phone

☐ Things to help the person function better and be less confused: hearing aids, eyeglasses, mobility aid (cane, walker, wheelchair)

☐ Medication list (or better yet the medications themselves, in a bag)

☐ Health insurance information

☐ Other health information (allergies, medical problems, names of doctors)

☐ Contact information for other family members

☐ Documentation of preferences of care (such as desire not to be resuscitated), and power of attorney

☐ Snacks and drinks for yourself and for the person with dementia

If Someone with Dementia Is in an Emergency Department and You Can't Be There:

- Arrange for a family member, home care worker, or neighbor to go with the person or meet them there and stay with them during the visit.

- Call before the person arrives. Explain why the person has been sent, that the person has dementia, and what the goals of care are. For instance, if you want the person home as soon as possible and don't want excessive testing done, you should communicate these wishes.

- Call every hour or so to ask how things are going. Be mindful that staff are busy, so keep the conversation short.

What You Can Do to Make the Emergency Visit Go Well

- Insist on staying with the person. If possible, have someone else along in case you need to step away.

- Always introduce yourself, explain the situation, and clarify goals for the visit. Say something like: "I'm his daughter; he's been living with me for three years, and I have power of attorney for health care decisions. My father may find it difficult to answer your questions—perhaps I can help?"

- Focus on what's different, when it started and how it's changing. For example, "this is NOT her typical state; normally she...."

- Tell staff what communication or care approach works best (for example, what name she responds best to), what distresses or makes her worse, and how to reduce her distress.

- Be prepared to repeat the same story to many health professionals, often across shifts.

- Keep your voice polite, calm, and reassuring—to model how to address a person with dementia.

- If you need to wait for a room or transport to a procedure, ask for a quiet place.

- Focus on soothing the person, rather than explaining the situation to them, especially if they don't have the ability to understand the situation.

- When it's discharge time, ask for details about what the health care providers think is going on and what they recommend.

- Don't leave without specific instructions and numbers to call if things change.

- When you leave, be sure you take home hearing aids, glasses, dentures, and other devices. These are expensive items that can be easy to lose.

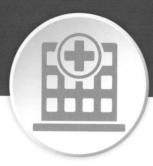

Hospital and After Hospital

Important! Caregivers must be a strong advocate for the person with dementia.

Hospitals Can be a Stressful Place for People with Dementia

A hospital can be a stressful, confusing place for persons with dementia. Hospitals are complex and can be difficult to navigate. There are increased risks of infection and medication errors. Miscommunication with staff is also common.

Don't be surprised if your relative is more agitated and/or confused in the hospital. It's also common to see the person's functional ability decline during and after a hospital stay.

Caregiver Checklist

Before Hospitalization

☐ Talk to a medical provider to understand why the person is being admitted, what tests or procedures will be done, the risks and benefits of these procedures, and the expected length of stay.

☐ Ask other family or friends to take turns staying in the hospital.

☐ Have advance directives prepared and placed in the person's medical record.

☐ Pack a hospitalization bag with the following:

- Medical information: insurance cards, medical history, medication list, advance directives.

- Supplies for you and the person you care for, such as changes of clothing, pictures from home, snacks, any personal care items you need.

- Comforting objects from home like pictures or a blanket.

☐ Bring hearing aids and glasses.

☐ Try to get a private room if possible.

During Hospitalization

☐ Talk to a medical provider daily about the plan for this hospital stay.

☐ Take notes when talking with doctors and nurses.

☐ Stay overnight or have someone else who knows the person stay with them.

☐ If family and friends offer to help, accept it.

☐ Tell medical providers about the needs of the person you care for.

☐ Wash your hands often and make sure visitors wash theirs too.

☐ Tell the staff if you see signs of pain, sleeping problems, or confusion.

☐ If the person is alert, keep their mind stimulated by talking with them.

Be prepared for early discharge and plan for it soon after arriving.

After Hospitalization: Discharge

☐ Discuss any limitations or specific desires you have concerning the person's care.

☐ Discuss rehabilitation with the provider. It may take place in the home, a rehabilitation facility, or nursing home.

☐ Make sure you have the following before leaving the hospital:

- A follow-up appointment with the person's primary care provider.

- A telephone number you can call at any time with questions.

- A list of potential problems to watch for.

- An updated medication list, with prescriptions for any new medications.

Common Concerns around Hospitalization of a Person with Dementia—What You Can Do

Concern	What You Can Do
Wandering	Tell the nurse if the person has wandered in the past. Talk about ways to keep the person from wandering.
Confusion and agitation	Make sure they have their glasses and hearing aids; remind them where they are; sit with the person and hold their hand; keep the room calm; make sure they sleep at night; avoid using bed restraints.
Pain	Talk with staff if you think the person is in pain and discuss treatment options. Watch for signs of pain.
Infections	Change the person's position often; wash your hands often. If the person has a urinary catheter, ask about an alternative.
Communicating with staff	Assign one family member to be the primary contact with staff; ask which nurse/provider you should direct questions to; prioritize the problems you want to discuss; take notes when you speak with a staff member; ask for educational materials; ask for a contact number before discharge, in case you have questions later.
Discharge	Discuss desires or concerns regarding care after discharge. If the person must go to a nursing home, ask about a special program or unit for dementia care. Make sure you understand any new diagnoses, the treatments received or needed, and what to watch for.
Rehabilitation	Pack comfortable and loose clothing for the person to use during rehab. Visit often and provide encouragement. Talk to the therapists and nurses.
Home health services	Consider what changes need to be made in the person's home, such as grab bars or a hospital bed. Get to know the person providing care. Try to be at home when the home health provider visits so you can learn from them.

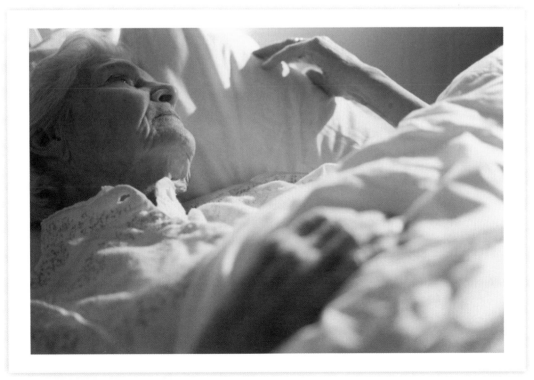

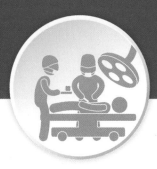

Surgery

Before and After Surgery Care

Surgery can be stressful and confusing for a person with dementia. Surgery in a person with dementia can create special challenges. Confusion (delirium) from stress, anesthesia, and pain medication can often occur. They may appear to get mentally worse after surgery. However, surgery is often necessary and can sometimes greatly improve the person's quality of life. Families need to decide if surgery is the right option and consider what the person would want.

What Will Surgery Be Like?

Step One: Medical Exam. Before surgery, the person will have a medical examination and undergo pre-surgery tests to determine if they are healthy enough for surgery.

Step Two: Pre-Operation (Day of Surgery). The person will go into a holding area where staff will confirm who they are and why they are there (for persons with dementia, a family member can do this). Then, they prepare the person for surgery. Anesthesia will be administered.

Step Three: Surgery. The length of the surgery will vary based on the type of procedure being done. It's best to have a friend or family member at the hospital during the whole procedure and recovery period.

Step Four: Post-surgery. The patient is moved to a post-operative care area where they are monitored. Once they have recovered from the anesthesia, the patient is transferred to a surgical ward or sent home.

Common Caregiver Concerns around Surgery in Persons with Dementia—What You Can Do

Concern	What You Can Do
Anesthesia	Ask the anesthesiologist what anesthesia will be used. Tell the surgical team if the person has had problems with anesthesia in the past. Give them a list of their medications including over-the-counter and natural/herbal remedies.
Confusion and agitation	Remind the patient that they had surgery and where they are. Keep the room calm and let them sleep. Keep the person busy when they are awake (such as by watching TV).
Pain	Talk with staff if you think the person is in pain, and discuss options to decrease pain.
Home care after surgery	Learn as much as you can from the medical staff about how to care for the person after surgery. Learn the common side effects and complications associated with the surgery. Encourage the amount and type of mobility the surgeon recommends.
Communicating with staff	Tell the nursing staff about the person's normal mental state and function. Tell staff about ways that work to calm the person down when they are agitated. If you are concerned about something, talk to the staff. Take notes when you speak with a staff member.
When you aren't there	See if another family member or friend can be with the person all the time; give the staff a phone number where they can reach you; check in regularly.

Caregiver Checklist

Before Surgery

- [ ] Get to know the physicians, including the surgeon, anesthesiologist, and medical doctor.

- [ ] Talk to a surgical team. Understand the risks and benefits of the surgery. **Questions to ask include:**

  - What is the procedure to be done, and who will be doing it?

  - When will the surgery take place, and how long will it take?

  - Where will the person go after surgery? Will they stay in the hospital or a rehabilitation facility or will they go home? How long is the recovery expected to last?

- [ ] Make sure the surgeon knows the person's medical history, medications, allergies, special diet requirements, and whether the person has family and friend support. Share any concerns you or the person with dementia have about the surgery.

- [ ] Ask what to bring prior to the surgery. Ask if any tests need to be done or changes made to their medication before surgery.

- [ ] Ask when the person will be discharged and where. If they are going home, ask what special equipment will be needed in the home, and how long it will be before the person is back to normal.

- [ ] Make sure the person doesn't eat or drink anything after midnight on the night before the surgery.

During Surgery

- [ ] Make sure you or someone else can be there for the whole surgery. If you cannot be there, make sure the staff have a phone number to reach you if needed during the surgery.

After Surgery

- [ ] Reach out to family and friends for support.

- [ ] If the person is going home, ask if a home health nurse and physical therapist can be provided.

- [ ] Keep an eye on the person's cognitive status, and look for signs of delirium, such as confusion and agitation. If you see signs of delirium, talk to the nurse or doctor.

- [ ] Make sure you have the following before leaving the hospital:

  - A follow-up appointment with the person's primary care provider.

  - A telephone number you can call at any time with questions.

  - A list of potential problems to watch for.

  - An updated medication list, with prescriptions for any new medications.

Don't be afraid to ask questions.

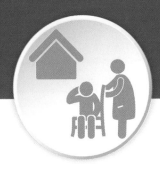

Paid In-Home Care

If the person with dementia is at home and you need assistance, consider hiring paid caregivers to come into the home. There are two main types of in-home care services: **home health care** and general **in-home services**.

Home health care is for people who have medical needs that require a nurse or other health care professional. Examples include after-hospital care, medication infusions, or physical therapy. These services may in part be covered by Medicare, Medicaid and/or private insurance.

General in-home services provide help with everyday activities and personal care, like bathing, dressing and preparing food. In-home caregivers can also ensure safety, provide socialization and companionship, and, when agreed upon, do household chores and shopping. These services are usually NOT covered by insurance, with the exception of Medicaid in some instances. The rest of this section discusses this type of in-home care.

In-home care can be provided by a certified nursing assistant (CNA), home health aide (HHA) or personal companion. CNAs have higher educational requirements and may be trained to do things like administer medications or provide wound care. In some states, home health aides are also trained to perform these types of duties.

You can hire in-home help through an agency or privately. There are pros and cons to each of these options.

Hiring through an agency:

Pros
- Many caregivers to choose from
- Available back-up if your caregiver is sick or has an emergency
- Agencies often take care of the taxes and liability/accident insurance
- Caregivers often have educational requirements like cardiopulmonary resuscitation (CPR) and first aid training
- Agencies often have a nurse supervising the caregivers

Cons
- Agencies are usually more expensive than hiring privately
- You may have less say regarding which caregiver is assigned

Hiring an individual who is not from an agency:

Pros
- A good option if you already know someone who is well recommended
- You will know who will be coming each time
- Usually less expensive than using an agency

Cons
- You may be responsible for costs if the caregiver is injured on the job
- In most cases, you'll be responsible for paying the caregiver's taxes and benefits, so consider consulting an accountant to determine your responsibilities
- No replacement if the caregiver is sick, on vacation or has an emergency

How to Address Concerns with Paid Caregivers

- Talk to the paid caregiver directly, in a calm and respectful manner, about the issue. Come up with a plan to resolve the issue.
- If this doesn't work and you've hired through an agency, talk to their supervisor.
- If the issue is important and not getting better despite good communication and problem solving, don't be afraid to fire the caregiver and move on.

Tips to Hire a Paid Caregiver Who is a Good Match

- Get recommendations from trusted family and friends.
- Interview potential caregivers.
- Observe how they interact with the person with dementia.
- Talk with at least two references.
- Ask for a 'trial' run of a week or two before signing an extended agreement.
- Be up-front, in writing, about expectations and duties. Include things that are not acceptable, like tardiness, smoking, bringing children to work, or non-emergency phone use. If working with an agency, insist on having input into the care plan. If you've hired an individual, insist on a formal, signed contract.
- Take time to train the caregiver. Provide notes about the habits, calming activities, likes, and dislikes of the person they will be caring for.
- Meet regularly to discuss problems, concerns and what's going well. If the person is doing a good job, tell them.

Suspected Abuse, Neglect or Theft by a Paid Caregiver

Rarely, paid caregivers may mistreat, abuse or neglect the person they're caring for, or steal from families.

For information on suspected abuse or neglect, including signs to look out for, see page 28.

To help protect your family from theft, hire only after you've talked to references for whom the person has worked (asking specifically if anything in the house disappeared) AND have conducted a criminal background check (or hired through an agency that performs background checks). If you suspect that theft has occurred, be cautious in accusing, as many people with dementia will move objects and not recall having done it. Speak to the caregiver using the tips provided on "how to address concerns."

Checklist of Tips for Caregivers

Questions to Ask an Agency

- ☐ Is your agency licensed? (required in certain states)
- ☐ Are your caregivers bonded and insured?
- ☐ How do you perform background checks? Do you check driving records?
- ☐ What are your caregivers' educational requirements?
- ☐ Are your caregivers screened for communicable diseases?
- ☐ Will you take care of all payroll paperwork?
- ☐ Can we interview potential caregivers and have input on who is assigned?
- ☐ Will we have the same caregiver each visit?
- ☐ What are the policies if our caregiver is unavailable? Will you provide an alternate? Is there an extra cost?
- ☐ How do you supervise caregivers? Will a nurse make occasional home visits? How often?
- ☐ What are the service agreement terms?
- ☐ What if I have a complaint about a caregiver?
- ☐ Can I have some references for your agency? For the caregiver we are assigned?

Questions to Ask an Individual Caregiver

- ☐ What is your caregiving experience? Do you have experience caring for someone with dementia?
- ☐ Why did you become a home caregiver?
- ☐ What is your training? Do you know CPR and first aid?
- ☐ Are you comfortable with (insert expected duties, like housework, helping someone who is anxious, cooking meals)?
- ☐ What times and days are you available and how many hours are you looking for?
- ☐ What are your holiday and time-off needs?
- ☐ What are your salary needs?
- ☐ Do you have a car? Are you comfortable driving with the care recipient?
- ☐ Do you have insurance?
- ☐ Are you bonded?
- ☐ Are you comfortable signing a care plan and/or contract?
- ☐ I will be doing a background check; is there anything I need to know?
- ☐ Can I have some references?

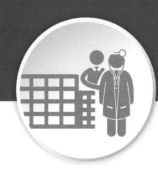

Residential, Long-Term Care

Nursing Home or Assisted Living

Residential long-term care settings, such as a nursing home or assisted living community, are a good alternative to in-home care for persons with dementia who need more care than family can provide. These settings provide assistance with activities such as bathing and managing chronic conditions, but they differ in the level of care provided and in their ability to care for persons with dementia, especially those with behavioral problems.

General Features of Assisted Living and Nursing Homes

	Assisted Living	Nursing Home
Clients	Often must do some things for themselves, such as eat and walk.	Need daily nursing services and/or can do little or nothing for themselves.
Services	Always includes 24-hour supervision, help with grooming and personal care, housekeeping, meals, social activities, and often at least some medication management. May include licensed nurse providers, on-site physician services, and some rehabilitative services.	Always includes 24-hour supervision, help with grooming and personal care, housekeeping, meals, activities, licensed nurses on-site 24/7, medication management, full rehabilitation services, and on-site doctor visits.
Cost	Varies widely by location and services provided. The national average is between $3,000 and $4,000 per month.	Varies by location, level of care and services provided. The national average is about $7,500 per month.
Payment Information	Usually self-pay. Medicare does not cover; Medicaid does in certain situations; some long-term care insurance provides coverage.	Self-pay, long-term care insurance, health insurance, Medicare, or Medicaid coverage based on the circumstance.

Choosing a Setting

- Look for a place close to the family and friends who will visit most often.
- If possible, have the person with dementia be part of the decision-making process.
- Determine whether the setting is able to meet the needs of the individual.
- Investigate the quality, reputation, or online ratings of the setting.
- Visit at different times of the day. Watch how staff interact with the residents and how involved the residents are in activities. You'll want a setting where staff are knowledgeable and caring, and where staff remain in their positions for a long time.

Moving In

- You may not want to involve the person in pre-move-in visits, as this can make them more anxious.
- If the person is angry or blames you—which is common—say that this is what has to be done for now (give a reason) and that you will help make it comfortable.
- Participate in the move-in and visit frequently.
- Leave visual and other reminders about having been there and when you will return.
- Verify the medication list with staff.

How to Work Well with Staff

- Share what you know, about your relative—likes and dislikes
- Treat staff with respect
- Give positive feedback
- Gently explain desired care (and when you don't see it, if that occurs)
- Recognize that you still remain a partner in caring for your relative, and in monitoring their condition and care.

What If I Have a Conflict with One or More Staff?

- Be aware that nursing assistants and other direct care providers have a hard job to do, with limited training, modest wages, and responsibility for many residents.
- Discuss problems calmly with the staff member involved or their supervisor. If that does not resolve the problem, speak with the nursing supervisor or the administrator.
- If your problem is still not resolved, start by contacting your local long-term care ombudsman. This office can guide you on how to file a complaint.

Memory Care Units

- "Dementia care" units or buildings exist in both assisted living communities and nursing homes.
- Research has **not** found better care or outcomes than in regular units. In both, quality depends on the leaders and the staff.
- A good memory care unit can provide these advantages: better security for people who wander, more dementia-specific activities and orientation, and less chance of overlooking the needs of someone who has dementia.

Common Concerns around Long-Term Care Settings—What You Can Do

Concern	What You Can Do
Feeling guilty or anxious	• Recognize that the majority of persons with dementia do eventually need residential care. Talk it over with family, friends, caregiver support groups, and/or professionals such as the Alzheimer's Association.
The person with dementia is unhappy or angry	• Remind yourself why you made the decision and why it was the right one. • Do your best to meet the person's need for love and attention. • Help the person adjust to his/her new living situation.
Abuse or theft	• If you suspect abuse, discuss it with the nursing director or administrator. • If you witness abuse, notify leadership and report it to the local adult protective services agency. For more information on abuse, see page 28. • Keep valuables at home and label dentures, eyeglasses and hearing aids.
The doctor is hard to see or contact	• Contact the health care provider by phone or speak to the provider's physician assistant or nurse practitioner.

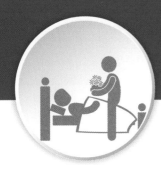

End-of-Life Care Services

Preparing Ahead for End-of-Life. The progression of dementia is unpredictable, so it's a good idea to consider preferences and make preparations ahead of time for end of life.

Palliative Care and Hospice. The term *palliative care* is used by the medical profession to talk about care that focuses on comfort rather than cure. Comfort care can be provided at any stage of chronic illness alongside treatments trying to cure the underlying disease. Palliative care for persons with dementia can be provided at home, a nursing home, a hospital, or specialized facilities, depending on family preferences and resources. Near the end of life, when comfort is the main goal, a special Medicare benefit called Hospice is often helpful.

Common End-of-Life Caregiver Questions

How do I prepare for the end of life?

- Communicate regularly with health care providers about the outlook and timetable for the illness.
- Prepare paperwork for medical professionals documenting wishes for treatment at the end of life. Each state in the country has a specific form for documenting this. Base these decisions on what the person has said or what you know generally about their preferences and wishes.
- Prepare finances, the will, and funeral arrangements in advance.

What are the signs that someone with dementia may be nearing death?

- Speaking few or no words, having bedsores/pressure ulcers, being unable to eat/swallow, repeated attacks of pneumonia or infection, and hospitalization for dehydration are more common as death is near.

What services are available for end-of-life care?

- Hospice and palliative care are the most common types of end-of-life care. With these end-of-life services, people are more likely to die in the location of their choice. Also, palliative care providers are better able to manage pain and prepare for end-of-life situations.
- Hospice can provide respite care for caregivers and counseling for a year after death.

Will Medicare or other insurance pay for hospice or palliative care?

- Medicare pays for certified Hospice services; to qualify, the health care provider must certify that the person is likely to die within six months.

How do most people with dementia die?

- In most cases, basic bodily functions slowly shut down. Pneumonia and dehydration are common conditions that contribute to or cause death.

Common Caregiver Concerns in Advanced Dementia – What You Can Do

Concern	What You Can Do
Trouble eating or swallowing	• If from weakness or fatigue, try feeding the person. • If from lack of appetite, try small amounts of favorite foods. • For coughing during swallowing, sit the person upright and have them tuck their chin in. • Be aware that force feeding, including feeding tubes, can cause more harm than good. Studies have shown that not eating and dehydration are not uncomfortable during the dying process.
Unable to communicate with the person	• Continue to talk to the person even if they seem non-responsive. • Communicate through touch.
Confusion and restlessness	• Make sure the person has their glasses and hearing aids; remind them where they are; sit with the person and hold their hand; keep the room calm.
Pain	• Stiff joints hurt, so when moving the person, do so slowly. • Drugs such as morphine can help decrease pain. • Use warm water or cool cloths to soothe muscles. • Consider alternative treatments such as massage, aromas, and music.
Caregiver fear, guilt, or depression	• Caregivers can experience many different feelings when someone they've lived with for years is dying. Common ones include fear of the dying process, grieving after the loss, and guilt about feeling relieved. • Understand that these are normal and may take a long time to work through. • Talk with family, a trusted friend, a clergyman or counselor, or Hospice staff.

What if the person wants to die at home?

• Both Hospice and palliative services can be provided at home.

• Ask about medications for pain, breathing problems, or other problems.

• Allow yourself to change your mind if things get too difficult.

• Accept help when offered.

If my relative has trouble communicating, how do I know if they are in pain?

• They may express their pain in some of the following ways: sighs, grunts, facial grimaces, agitation or aggression, abnormal body positions or guarding the part that hurts, or unusual descriptions like "not right" or "tight" if they can still communicate through words.

What should I do when I am with someone who is dying?

• Hold hands or provide other soothing touch.

• Talk to them, even if they are non-responsive.

• Play familiar music.

I send the questions I have
for the doctor by e-mail before our
appointment. Thinking about the
questions in advance really helps,
when you're not under the stress of
making it through the appointment.

— *Kathy L., caregiver*

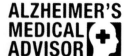

Useful Information to Have on Hand: Recording Sheets

It can be especially challenging communicating your concerns to health care providers when caring for a person with dementia.

The following pages are for you to fill out before you call or see a health care provider. You may wish to remove them from this book or (better yet) make multiple photocopies. By gathering this information in advance, you'll likely find the call or visit more productive and helpful.

Information to Gather Before Calling or Seeing a Health Care Provider

This form can help you organize and communicate a new concern to the health care provider. It is especially useful if there are multiple caregivers sharing caregiving responsibilities.

Personal Health Record

This form is a handy record of the person's family contacts, physicians, medical problems, medicines, allergies and insurance. Almost all visits require some or all of this information.

Vital Signs Recording Sheet

Use this sheet to record the person's vital signs regularly, so that you'll get to know their usual measurements. If you have concerns, bring this sheet with you during provider visits and make additional copies for future use.

Information to Gather Before Calling or Seeing a Health Care Provider about a New or Worsening Medical or Behavioral Issue

Patient's Name: _____ Date of Birth:_____/_____/_____
                                                                month   day   year

Describe the problem in detail. Include when it started, what you think might be causing the problem, and any things you have done to help relieve the problem.

_____

_____

_____

Does the person NOW appear normal or back to normal? ☐ yes ☐ no ☐ not sure
If no or not sure, what is different? _____

_____

Vital signs (record all that are available)	☐ Heart rate (pulse):_____ beats per minute
	☐ Breathing (respiratory) rate:_____breaths per minute
	☐ Temperature:_____degrees ☐ Fahrenheit ☐ Celsius
	☐ Blood pressure: _____ / _____

Provide a little background about the person's dementia. Is it (check one):
☐ very early   ☐ mild   ☐ moderate   ☐ severe   ☐ very severe

To the best of your knowledge, what is the diagnosis: _____

Has the person started, stopped, or changed a medication within the last two weeks?
☐ don't know   ☐ no   ☐ yes **If yes** ⟶ What was the change? _____

If there is anything about the person's medical history that you feel may be especially relevant to this problem, list and describe it here._____

_____

_____

Is there anything in particular that you are worried about or want to know? ☐ yes ☐ no

If yes, please explain: _____

Name of Person Completing Form: _____ Phone ( ) _____-_____

Relationship to the person with dementia: _____

Today's date: ____/____/_____ Time completed: ____:_____ AM PM (circle one)

When talking with a health professional, have a list of the person's current medications and allergies, plus the name and phone number of their pharmacy.

Personal Health Record

Patient's Name: _____ Date of Birth:_____/_____/_____

Family/Friends to Contact in Emergency

1. **Name:**_____

   Relationship:_____

   Home Phone:_____

   Cell Phone:_____

2. **Name:**_____

   Relationship:_____

   Home Phone:_____

   Cell Phone:_____

Main Physicians and/or Care Agencies:

1. **Name:**_____

   Specialty:_____

   Phone:_____

2. **Name:**_____

   Specialty:_____

   Phone:_____

Hospital of Choice:_____

   Location:_____

Care Preferences (check all that apply):

☐ Do everything, including resuscitation
  and breathing tube

☐ Has legal document stating preferences for limiting
  care (e.g., living will or DNR)

☐ Power of attorney for health care decisions:

   Name: _____

   Phone: _____

☐ Other: _____

Main Medical Problems

1. _____

2. _____

3. _____

4. _____

5. _____

6. _____

Current Medications last updated ___/___/20____

Name	Dose/Times per day
_____	_____
_____	_____
_____	_____
_____	_____
_____	_____
_____	_____
_____	_____
_____	_____
_____	_____
_____	_____

Medication Allergies:

Medication Name	Type of Reaction
_____	_____
_____	_____

Recent Immunizations [recommended frequency]:

☐ **Flu** [every year]   Last received: _____

☐ **Pneumonia** [once]   Last received:_____

☐ **Shingles** [once]   Last received: _____

☐ **Tetanus** [every 10 yrs] Last received: _____

Insurance Information (check all that apply and provide policy numbers):

☐ **Medicare Part A:**
   Policy #_____

☐ **Medicare Part B:**
   Policy # _____

☐ **Private Medicare Supplement**
   Company:_____
   Policy # _____

☐ **Medicaid**
   Policy #_____

☐ **Veterans:**
   Policy # _____

☐ **Private Insurance:**
   Company: _____
   Policy # _____

Vital Signs Recording Sheet

Date	Time	Pulse	Breathing Rate	Temperature	Blood Pressure
____/____/_____	____:____ AM PM	_____	_____	_____	_____/_____
____/____/_____	____:____ AM PM	_____	_____	_____	_____/_____
____/____/_____	____:____ AM PM	_____	_____	_____	_____/_____
____/____/_____	____:____ AM PM	_____	_____	_____	_____/_____
____/____/_____	____:____ AM PM	_____	_____	_____	_____/_____
____/____/_____	____:____ AM PM	_____	_____	_____	_____/_____
____/____/_____	____:____ AM PM	_____	_____	_____	_____/_____
____/____/_____	____:____ AM PM	_____	_____	_____	_____/_____
____/____/_____	____:____ AM PM	_____	_____	_____	_____/_____
____/____/_____	____:____ AM PM	_____	_____	_____	_____/_____
____/____/_____	____:____ AM PM	_____	_____	_____	_____/_____
____/____/_____	____:____ AM PM	_____	_____	_____	_____/_____
____/____/_____	____:____ AM PM	_____	_____	_____	_____/_____
____/____/_____	____:____ AM PM	_____	_____	_____	_____/_____
____/____/_____	____:____ AM PM	_____	_____	_____	_____/_____
____/____/_____	____:____ AM PM	_____	_____	_____	_____/_____
____/____/_____	____:____ AM PM	_____	_____	_____	_____/_____
____/____/_____	____:____ AM PM	_____	_____	_____	_____/_____
____/____/_____	____:____ AM PM	_____	_____	_____	_____/_____
____/____/_____	____:____ AM PM	_____	_____	_____	_____/_____
____/____/_____	____:____ AM PM	_____	_____	_____	_____/_____
____/____/_____	____:____ AM PM	_____	_____	_____	_____/_____
____/____/_____	____:____ AM PM	_____	_____	_____	_____/_____

Vital signs should be taken while the person is resting and relaxed. "Normal" varies depending on the person, time of day, and activity. Normal values for older persons are typically within the following ranges (with a little variation above and below for some people): 55-80 beats per minute for pulse, 10-20 breaths per minute for breathing rate, 96.4-99.0° F for temperature by mouth, and 100-150 / 50-90 for blood pressure.

INDEX